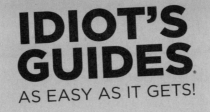

IDIOT'S GUIDES.
AS EASY AS IT GETS!

Healthy Gut Diet

by S. Jane Gari and Wendie Schneider, RDN, LD, MBA

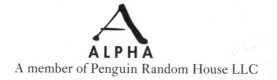

ALPHA
A member of Penguin Random House LLC

Publisher: Mike Sanders
Associate Publisher: Billy Fields
Acquisitions Editor: Jan Lynn
Development Editor: Donna Wright
Cover Designer: Lindsay Dobbs
Book Designer: William Thomas
Compositor: Ayanna Lacey
Proofreader: Cate Schwenk
Indexer: Tonya Heard

First American Edition, 2016
Published in the United States by DK Publishing
6081 E. 82nd Street, Indianapolis, Indiana 46250

Copyright © 2016 Dorling Kindersley Limited
A Penguin Random House Company
16 17 18 19   10 9 8 7 6 5 4 3 2 1
001-290405-MAY2016

Published in the United States by Dorling Kindersley Limited.

IDIOT'S GUIDES and Design are trademarks of Penguin Random House LLC

ISBN: 9781615648917
Library of Congress Catalog Card Number: 2015951837

Note: This publication contains the opinions and ideas of its author(s). It is intended
to provide helpful and informative material on the subject matter covered. It is sold
with the understanding that the author(s) and publisher are not engaged in rendering
professional services in the book. If the reader requires personal assistance or
advice, a competent professional should be consulted, especially if the reader has a
preexisting medical condition or is pregnant or nursing. The author(s) and publisher
specifically disclaim any responsibility for any liability, loss, or risk, personal or
otherwise, which is incurred as a consequence, directly or indirectly, of the use and
application of any of the contents of this book.

Trademarks: All terms mentioned in this book that are known to be or are suspected
of being trademarks or service marks have been appropriately capitalized. Alpha
Books, DK, and Penguin Random House LLC cannot attest to the accuracy of this
information. Use of a term in this book should not be regarded as affecting the
validity of any trademark or service mark.

DK books are available at special discounts when purchased in bulk for sales
promotions, premiums, fund-raising, or educational use. For details, contact: DK
Publishing Special Markets, 345 Hudson Street, New York, New York 10014 or
SpecialSales@dk.com.

Printed and bound in the United States of America

idiotsguides.com

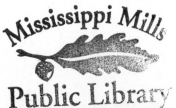

Contents

Introduction

"You are what you eat." We've all heard this, but what does that really mean? Simply put, the most important factor in your overall health is the food you put into your body. The interactions between food and parts of your digestive system, your "gut," determine the strength of your immunity, the diseases your body will develop, and even your learning potential and emotional well-being.

In this book, you learn how problems in the gut can affect your entire body. More importantly, you educate yourself about body processes and food preparation to lessen, heal, and even prevent gut problems. What happens along this tract is paramount to your overall health. The best news? Your eating and lifestyle choices can influence its health. You control what goes into your body and troubleshoot how it reacts to certain foods. "Listen to your gut" is advice you should take literally.

According to a survey conducted by a major pharmaceutical company (AbbVie), 74 percent of Americans live with persistent gastrointestinal ("gut") problems, and almost half of them never report these issues to a doctor. Embarrassment and fear often prevent people from seeking help. By learning the science governing your gut, you can address the underlying conditions that cause digestive discomfort and disease.

While addressing gastrointestinal concerns sometimes means turning to the medical community, doctors are often undereducated about nutrition and how to cultivate a healthy gut. A deficit in nutritional education has governed conventional medicine for decades, and from some doctors' perspective, drugs are the main means of combatting illness. Prevention is given far less attention. But there is reason for optimism as more and more doctors adopt an integrative approach to the patient, including nutritional counseling. Still, it's important that you take charge of your health by seeking professional nutritional advice and educating yourself about the inner workings of your gut.

Prevention of any illness starts in the immune system. What does that have to do with your gut? An astounding 70 to 80 percent of your body's immune cells live there. Gut issues can cause immune responses and chemical imbalances that lead to diabetes, chronic fatigue, autoimmune disease, skin disorders, inflammation, allergies, and respiratory disease. New studies demonstrate how the quality of bacteria living in your gut can have a serious impact on your overall physical and mental well-being. And you have complete control over the most important contributing factor to a healthy gut: your diet.

The major challenge in the quest for gut health? "Healthy" foods are sometimes hard to define as our food supply has drifted away from whole foods and toward processed, foodlike products that are difficult to digest and actually cause damage to the intestinal lining. Many foods cause chemical reactions that, over time, can literally create gaps and holes in the walls of the intestine, referred to as intestinal hyperpermeability or "leaky gut syndrome." Abnormally large spaces in the intestinal lining allow bad bacteria to get out of control and permit undigested bits of food to get into your bloodstream, which can cause your immune system to get out of whack.

To some people, the diet guidelines suggested in this book might sound too drastic or different from what they're accustomed to eating. Only you can decide the pace and extent of your commitment. Some folks like to dive into lifestyle changes head first to achieve optimal results. Most people achieve long-term success by integrating a series of small to moderate changes over time. But rest assured—every step you take toward gut health will have positive benefits.

In this book, we explain how you can improve your overall health and even prevent and mitigate disease by making better nutritional and lifestyle choices. We present and evaluate the science available on the topic so you can take more control of your health by making the best choices for your own healthy gut.

How This Book Is Organized

To make this book easy to use, we divided the information into five sections:

Part 1, Getting to Know Your Gut, explains the workings of your digestive system, the parts of the body that make up the gut, and what role they play. We also help you determine if your gut function and health is normal and when to be concerned. We introduce you to the microscopic organisms that call your gut home, and you learn how to nourish them so they help you build immunity and absorb nutrients. We also discuss how damaged guts develop and ways to get diagnosed. You learn how to assemble an appropriate team of health practitioners to help you achieve optimal gut health safely and effectively, and we provide a review of specific medical tests to request for food sensitivity panels and bacteria overgrowth. Finally, we share the foods that most commonly trigger negative gut reactions like gluten, dairy, and refined sugars.

Part 2, Understanding Leaky Gut Syndrome, explains how the typical diet and modern lifestyle choices can lead to abnormally large gaps in the lining of your gut, or leaky gut syndrome. We look at the history of the syndrome and the consensus of modern science on the subject. More importantly, we show you how to take advantage of this science to achieve optimal health. We also examine the specifics of how intestinal hyperpermeability can lead to physical and mental health issues and share which foods and medications can aggravate the gut so you can limit your use or even avoid them altogether.

Part 3, Repairing the Leaks, gives you the basics of how to heal your gut through diet. You learn how to eliminate "gut-wrenching" foods, choose foods your gut bacteria love, and safely detox your digestive system. We provide guidelines for tracking your progress with food diaries and applying the results of food sensitivity panels and share lists of healthy foods and supplements that aid in repairing a damaged gut and promote optimal gut health. You also learn how to read your metabolism, understand why you should avoid foods that trigger harmful reactions in your system, and learn to replace your favorite trigger foods with healthy alternatives. We also discuss other lifestyle choices that help your gut perform optimally and offer tips to manage common household toxins and exercise suggestions. We compare the most prominent diets whose guidelines promise to heal the gut and give you the consensus of the best advice backed by science.

Part 4, Living the Healthy Gut Diet, navigates the transition to healthier eating with grocery lists, meal-planning guides, and recipes. We even account for the times when sticking to a dietary regimen is challenged the most—during travel and holiday celebrations. We also provide tools to help you overcome the enemies of success: temptation, negativity, and daily stress. You learn to combat these enemies with knowledge, exercise, meditation, and preparedness.

Part 5, Finding a Healthy Gut Balance, discusses what to expect when you launch your healthy gut diet. We cover what's normal and offer advice that helps you get back on track if and when you experience setbacks. We also explain the long-term benefits of sticking to the diet and how to transition back to the typical diet if you choose.

Extras

Sprinkled throughout this book you find little nuggets of information of interest as you read.

ASK THE EXPERTS

In these sidebars, medical doctors, dieticians, and nutritionists weigh in on how to achieve the healthy gut lifestyle.

DEFINITION

These sidebars contain definitions related to gut health.

GUT WISE

Follow these tips and suggestions to help you succeed with the healthy gut diet.

YOU ARE WHAT YOU EAT

Here, you find interesting food facts to help you with gut health.

We also share Success Stories throughout that offer real-life accounts of people who took charge of their gut health.

Acknowledgments

Michelle Johnson, of Inklings Literary, is my outstanding literary agent whose encouragement and confidence made my involvement in this project possible. I would also like to thank Dr. Mark Houllif of Consultative Health and Nutrition in Brooklyn, New York; his guidance enabled my recovery and helped me reclaim a healthy life. Thank you also to Kristen Tice-Ziesmer, RD, CSSD, of Elite Nutrition and Performance in Columbia, South Carolina, for her contributions. A special thank you to my co-author, Wendie Schneider, for agreeing to partner on this project and keep me honest. Her philosophy, background, and expertise were paramount to the completion of this book. To my family and friends, thank you for your patience while I navigated many trials and errors in my quest for optimal gut health. I'm so grateful to my friend Greg Oaks who introduced me to the work of Dr. Joel Fuhrman, which was the impetus for my nutritional research and ultimate recovery. To my husband especially, thank you for never losing faith in me and shoring me up all these years. —Jane

I want to thank my co-author, Jane Gari, for the time, hard work, and dedication she put into this book. To my family and friends, thank you for supporting me in everything I do. You are all a continual source of encouragement for me. Special thanks goes out to one of my very best friends, mentor, and business partner, Andrew Brandenburg, who gives me creative inspiration when I get stuck and is the most patient person I know. To all my clients that have contributed to this book through examples, questions, suggestions, and experiences through the years, working with you has been a pleasure and a gift to me. —Wendie

Getting to Know Your Gut

Do you ever stop to think about what happens in your body as you're eating? In Part 1, we take a journey through the key parts of your digestive tract. You learn how to tell if they're in top shape or not by comparing how your digestive history compares to normal ranges of gastrointestinal function.

This part also defines the parts that make up your gut and how it interacts with other parts of your body. Discover the amazing world of bacteria that live inside of you. They are an ecosystem unto themselves, but they communicate with your body, helping you digest food and defend against illness. Learn how keeping them happy helps these bacteria work for you.

Finally, Part 1 explores the connections between your gut and overall health. It gives advice about how to take control of your gut health by partnering with health practitioners.

Gut Basics

Your gut, or digestive system, is a key player in your overall health. You need to take in food to produce the energy your body needs to function. Now more than ever science can explain the interactions between your gut and the rest of your body. Understanding the inner workings of your gut can prevent, mitigate and, in some cases, reverse many diseases.

In this chapter, you learn the basic parts of your gut and how they function. We break down the new science that explores the connections between the gut and the brain.

In This Chapter

- Your gut's overall functions
- The different parts of your digestive system
- Nutrient absorption and distribution
- How your gut communicates with the rest of your body
- Your "second brain" in your digestive system

What Is Your Gut's Job?

Your gut, or the tube that begins at your mouth and ends at your anus, has many functions. It breaks down food into nutrients and then absorbs those nutrients so the body can use them. After processing everything useful the food has to offer, the gut disposes of the waste.

The gut also helps regulate your immune system. The majority of the immune cells in your body lie in your gut. The cells and helpful bacteria in your digestive system provide a first line of defense against invaders that hitch a ride into your body on the food you eat. The journey through your gut is a fascinating ride.

Food Digestion

Digestion is gut job number one. Digestion is the bodily process that converts food into usable energy for your body's cells. The cells that make up your body can't get the *nutrients* they need from food in its original state. Digestion essentially sucks the best and simplest parts out of food and shrinks and distills them into pieces so small, they can be absorbed by the cells and used for your bodily functions.

Cells are the building blocks of life. Similarly structured cells in your body combine to form tissues. Those tissues combine to form organs, and organs that work together for certain specialized functions form systems. When we refer to "the gut," we are talking about some of the more prominent players in your digestive system. Your digestive system is in charge of transforming food into small energy packages your body can use. You need this process to survive.

Digestion involves muscles and *enzymes* and the cooperation of multiple organs and systems. This process is both mechanical and chemical. This makes it sound as if there are engines and drug labs in your body. While that's not exactly the case, those are pretty good analogies.

Mechanical literally means having to do with physical forces. And there are physical forces at work in digestion. Food is being chewed and then swallowed. In your stomach, food is churned around for hours at a time, another mechanical action. *Peristalsis,* the series of internal muscular contractions that move food throughout your digestive tract, is a very mechanical process.

> **DEFINITION**
>
> **Nutrients** are substances containing nourishment crucial for maintaining life. A substance made by a living thing that aids in chemical reactions like those involved in digestion is called an **enzyme.** The series of involuntary muscular contractions along the gastrointestinal tract, called **peristalsis,** work to propel the contents of the gut forward.

The chemical part of digestion involves digestive juices and enzymes. These substances cause chemical reactions that break down the food particles into nutrients that can then be absorbed by your body. The chemistry of digestion happens in conjunction with all the mechanical action. Different parts of the digestive tract release chemical compounds that help turn whole foods into small nutrients.

Nutrient Absorption

Your gut's job is to obtain nutrients from the food, absorb them and then deliver them to other systems in the body. *Nutrients* are substances containing nourishment necessary to sustain and maintain life. These substances are the smallest useful components in food. They're necessary to keep your body working properly.

So how does your body absorb and use nutrients? It depends on what kind of nutrient it is. Nutrients are divided into two main categories: macronutrients and micronutrients.

Macronutrients include carbohydrates, proteins, and fats; these can be broken down relatively quickly and provide more direct energy to the body.

 YOU ARE WHAT YOU EAT

Why do we demonize carbs? The secret is moderation. Here's the skinny on carbs: your brain uses about 60 percent of the carbs you eat when you just relax! Muscle has the unique ability to store carbohydrates for energy later in a form called glycogen. Fat cells store excess carbs for later use as triglycerides. The liver is the master of metabolism. This guy uses stored glucose (from carbs) for energy to process and metabolize literally everything we put into our body.

Micronutrients include vitamins and minerals. These substances act as catalysts in the chemical reactions involved in releasing energy from macronutrients. Like a lot of substances in the body, these two types of nutrients need to have a symbiotic relationship. In other words, they should work happily together.

Almost all nutrient absorption happens in your small intestine. The integrity or "wholeness" of the lining in your small intestine is one of the most important elements of gut health. Nutrients pass through the walls of your small intestine and enter your *circulatory system,* where they are transported to the rest of your body by way of your *cardiovascular* or *lymphatic systems.* In other words, sometimes nutrients are sent right into your bloodstream; at other times, the nutrients are released via other pathways in your body that carry fluid and cells that aid in your body's natural immunity and defense against disease.

> **DEFINITION**
>
> The **circulatory system** is responsible for moving blood and lymph through the body; it is made up of the **cardiovascular system,** which includes the heart, arteries, capillaries, and veins, and the **lymphatic system,** which consists of lymphatic vessels and glands. Together, these two branches of the circulatory system regulate protein levels in the blood, regulate pH levels, filter out bacteria, and ward off disease and infection.

The two main avenues nutrients take through the intestinal wall are called active and passive transport. In passive transport, nutrients can move from the intestine to the bloodstream with very little cellular energy required—it's an easy "downhill" path. All vitamins pass into your bloodstream via passive transport. In active transport, the nutrients need what's referred to as a "helper" or "carrier" molecule—much like pushing a car uphill. These helper molecules are usually enzymes that aid the passage of the nutrient directly into general circulation in the body. Both of these avenues help deliver nutrients to all the other systems in your body.

Waste Disposal

As embarrassing as it may seem, waste products of digestion are some of the lowest common denominators of the human experience. It's a necessary fact of life. Understanding the mechanics of human waste elimination will give you insight about what is normal so you're better equipped to identify and then deal with problems if they arise.

After parts of your digestive system have worked in conjunction with your circulatory system to break down food and absorb nutrients, there is some material leftover. This undigested, unused food residue moves into your large intestine. Bacteria that live in your large intestine actually turn this residue into feces by removing the water from it. Then the feces makes its way through the rectum and out of your anus so you can eliminate that waste.

So where does urine come from? The *urinary system* takes care of that. Your kidneys work like a filter. As blood passes through your kidneys, water and other important substances, like nutrients, are returned to your bloodstream. Then the liquid waste leaves your kidneys via pathways calls ureters, which lead to the urinary bladder. That waste, called urine, then leaves your bladder through your urethra.

> **GUT WISE**
>
> Remember, if you are not drinking enough water, it will be much harder for your body to combat everyday stress, fight off fatigue, digest foods, and keep up your metabolism. In general, you need 8 to 10 cups per day. This can change depending on how much you sweat and/or exercise. One rule of thumb is to drink until your pee is clear. That is the physical signal you are fully hydrated.

Immunity

Approximately 70 percent of your body's immune cells are located in your digestive system. The largest concentration of these cells connect to the gut mucosa, which is the lining of your intestinal wall. The gut mucosa help manufacture *lymphocytes*, which are a kind of white blood cell that helps attack harmful invaders in your body. The first point of contact between you and illness is often your gut. When bad bacteria and viruses are introduced to your body through your gut, a healthy immune system will be able to avoid getting sick.

In addition to immune cells, your gut is home to trillions of good bacteria that play a key role in the healthy functioning of your immune system. Ideally, these bacteria work in a symbiotic relationship with your immune cells, and the lining of the intestine, to keep everything running smoothly in the gut and to keep out bad invaders, like *pathogens*. Recent science has uncovered the links between diet, gut bacteria, and immunity.

DEFINITION

Your **urinary system** consists of your kidneys, ureters, urinary bladder, and urethra; the function of the system is to filter, collect, and eliminate waste products from your blood in the form of urine. **Lymphocytes** are white blood cells of the immune system that attack foreign invaders throughout your body. A **pathogen** is a substance or small organism that causes disease in another larger organism (living thing).

Your diet directly influences the bacteria population in your gut. The wrong kind of food can encourage an overgrowth of bad bacteria that crowd out the healthy kind. These imbalances compromise the ability of your gut to create immune cells.

Over time, imbalance in the gut can also compromise the capability of your intestinal lining to keep bad bacteria, undigested food particles, and pathogens from passing into your circulatory and lymphatic systems. This scenario is often referred to as "leaky gut" or "leaky gut syndrome." Leaky gut can lead to immune dysfunction that can give rise to food intolerances, allergies, autoimmune disorders, and inflammatory conditions. This is why it's extremely important to take care of your gut by taking in the right kind of fuel—healthy food.

The Parts of Your Gut

Your digestive system is impressive. If you could remove all the parts of its "tube," even uncoiling the mazelike structures of your small intestine, and lay them all flat, the average adult's *gastrointestinal tract* would stretch out for about 30 feet. This amazing tube works in conjunction with your nervous system, circulatory system, and the other organs in your digestive system.

When you are hungry, or smell something delicious cooking on the stove, or even see a commercial for something appetizing, your *central nervous system* (CNS) starts sending signals to your gastrointestinal tract to start secreting enzymes and hormones that will help break down the food your body is anticipating. Once that food is introduced to your gut, the different components go to work—highly specialized work.

Your GI Tract

Your gut is also called your gastrointestinal tract (GI tract). In essence, your gut is a tube that begins in your mouth and ends with your anus. Its main job is to break down foods through digestion, absorb nutrients, and prevent harmful bacteria from entering other organs.

Once you start chewing and swallowing food, the secretions along your gut increase and the muscular contractions of peristalsis begin. After your stomach is done churning around, food residue moves through your small and large intestines. Finally, after every last ounce of nutrients can be absorbed from the food, the remaining residue is eliminating via your anus.

Now let's look at how each part of your gut accomplishes this process.

Your Mouth, Tongue, and Salivary Glands

Your central nervous system sends signals to the *salivary glands* in your mouth to produce and secrete more *saliva*. So yes, food can literally, "make your mouth water." Once the food hits your tongue and your taste buds get in on the action, your salivary glands produce even more saliva. Saliva is magical stuff. It contains an important enzyme called amylase that starts the breakdown of starches you eat and converts them into simpler sugars. The main job of breaking down starches is done in your small intestine, but your mouth gets things started. About 30 percent of starch digestion happens in your mouth.

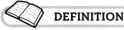 **DEFINITION**

> The line of tubular tissues and organs responsible for digesting food that extends from your mouth to your anus is called the **gastrointestinal tract.** Your **central nervous system** is made of your brain and spinal cord. **Salivary glands** are structures in your mouth that secrete **saliva,** a watery substance rich in enzymes that help break down starches in the first stage of digestion.

Your teeth, aided by your tongue, push food around and grind it down. This mechanical process literally breaks down food into smaller pieces and causes even more saliva to be secreted. The softer mass of food in your mouth after chewing is now ready for the next stop in your gut.

Your Pharynx and Esophagus

Pharynx is just the medical term for your throat. It receives the food after you've chewed it up, and your tongue and the roof of your mouth help push it back there. Your pharynx branches off into the trachea, which leads to your lungs, and your esophagus, which leads to your stomach. Every once in a while, food doesn't go directly to your stomach—hence the origin of coughing people gasping the phrase, "it went down the wrong pipe." In serious circumstances, food trapped in the trachea can block off a person's air supply and cause them to choke. Luckily, the act of swallowing that takes place in your throat is a partially voluntary action, so take your time and chew your food carefully.

Ideally, the act of swallowing temporarily closes your trachea so food is goes into your esophagus. Your esophagus is lined with muscles that contract and send food toward your stomach.

Your Stomach

Right before the entrance to your stomach is a sphincter, a ring-shaped muscle, known as the *lower esophageal sphincter* (*LES*). This muscle is the gatekeeper to your stomach. It opens to let food in and should close shut to keep food in your stomach with its stronger enzymes and gastric juices like hydrochloric acid.

Your stomach is a J-shaped, saclike organ. Its lining is full of muscles that grind food to a liquid or paste consistency. Your stomach lining is also home to receptor cells that send additional signals to more glands to release even more gastric juices. The muscle contractions of the stomach walls and the stomach juices all help break down food even further before sending it through another sphincter (the *pyloric sphincter*) that leads to your small intestine.

Your Small Intestine

Your small intestine is the MVP of your gut. The small intestine accounts for 20 of the 30 feet of an average adult GI tract. The majority of digestion, and nearly all nutrient absorption, happen in your small intestine.

Like other parts of your GI tract, your small intestine relies on the secretion of substances, such as enzymes, to further break down food particles. Two other digestive organs that are not part of the GI tract, the pancreas and gallbladder, lend their secretions to your small intestine via specialized ducts, or pathways that lead from these organs to your small intestine. *Enterocytes,* the cells of the small intestine's surface, also secrete their own enzymes.

The ring-shaped muscle that serves as the pathway from your esophagus into your stomach is known as the **lower esophageal sphincter (LES).** The **pyloric sphincter** is another ring-shaped muscle that serves as the pathway from your stomach into the first section of your small intestine known as the duodenum. **Enterocytes** are the epithelial cells (single-layer surface cells) of the small intestine.

The internal walls of your small intestine boast some pretty cool structures called villi. These fingerlike villi are covered by even smaller microvilli. The purpose of these structures is to increase the surface area of your intestine—more surface area equals more nutrient absorption. The villi and microvilli act like little tentacles that trap the nutrients in your intestine and pull the nutrients directly to the enterocytes of the intestinal surface.

The enterocytes are responsible for releasing the nutrients into your circulatory system via the passive and transport mechanisms discussed earlier. These "delivery systems" transport nutrients to the rest of your body. All the functions of the small intestine are affected by the health of the bacteria that live there. (We discuss those bacteria in more detail in Chapter 3.)

Your Large Intestine and Rectum

Your large intestine is much shorter than your small intestine; it's only about 5 feet long. However, the inside of this other tubular organ is much wider. There are no villi or microvilli here. The main job of the large intestine is to absorb potassium and sodium and any remaining water from the food residue passing through it. There are also bacteria in the large intestine that assist in this last stage of digestion and help form stools (feces).

Muscles in your large intestine move the feces toward the rectum causing the rectal walls to stretch. Receptors in the rectal walls communicate with your spinal cord to increase pressure on the first sphincter of the anus. This is when you get that urge to go. Thankfully, the second sphincter of the anus is under voluntary control, or at least it is under the best of circumstances. Controlling that second sphincter is what young children learn to do during potty-training. Healthy people can control whether or not they open their bowels to let out feces.

How Your Gut Works with Your Brain

Your brain is an amazing organ that houses memory and allows you to experience emotion. It also sends signals to other body systems, including your digestive system, to prime those systems to perform their functions properly. Receptors and nerves in the gut and the brain allow them to communicate with each other. The pathway of nerves that connect your gut and your brain involves and is influenced by not only digestion but also emotions. The science shows those gut feelings you have are very real after all.

Digestion Begins in Your Head

Your brain processes all your five senses, and taste and smell are what combine to allow you to experience the actual flavors of food. While this is impressive, it can cause some complications when it comes to eating. Hunger and thirst are physical factors that drive the need to eat. You literally feel these factors in various parts of your gut. But what and how you actually eat is influenced by other psychological factors that are more nuanced.

Sometimes you might eat when you're not hungry, out of boredom or sadness. Sometimes certain flavors activate pleasure sensors in the brain, and you keep eating more just for pleasure rather than need. Then, when you want to repeat that experience, you choose foods that satisfy flavor preferences. Flavor can be an overwhelming force. Your pleasure-seeking impulses are not always in line with sound nutritional choices. This is a conflict at the root of many gut health issues. What you crave isn't always best for you.

GUT WISE

When you are hungry, you might actually be thirsty? Try this: when you are hungry, drink 8 ounces of water and wait 10 to 15 minutes before taking a gut check. Listen to your hunger cues before grabbing food and just eating on autopilot.

Your Vagus Nerve

Many nerves extend from your brain to other parts of your body. The *vagus nerve* is the longest of these nerves and branches out to multiple organs in your chest and abdomen. It's a communication highway between your gut and brain.

Before you even put food in your mouth, your brain releases special chemical messengers, called *neurotransmitters,* to your gut via the vagus nerve. These chemical messengers travel along this pathway, sending signals for your gut to secrete saliva and gastric juices in preparation to receive food. The vagus nerve also aids in the impulse to swallow and the muscle contractions that push food along your GI tract during peristalsis. This same nerve pathway lets your brain know your stomach is full, so you'll stop eating.

> **GUT WISE**
>
> Eating slowly can help you lose weight and prevent overeating. It takes about 20 min-
> utes for the signals to travel from your gut to your brain and register that you're full.
> Giving your body time to send and receive those signals eases bloating and prevents
> you from feeling stuffed. And when you chew raw vegetables until they feel liquefied
> in your mouth, you've cracked open all the plant cells. This increases your chances of
> getting every nutrient that food has to offer.

Because your vagus nerve also runs through your chest, it influences your heart rate, blood pressure, and breathing. Just as the pleasure sensors in your brain can affect your eating choices, the
vagus nerve can have an impact on how you respond to stress. When you're facing an emotionally taxing situation or a stressful scenario, your vagus never can become overstimulated. This
is what causes "butterflies in the stomach" when you're nervous or frightened, or a "gut feeling"
when you're anxious or apprehensive about an unknown outcome. The vagus nerve helps activate
the "fight or flight" response that reduces the production of digestive juices and limits the flow of
blood to your gut. This why when you're overly nervous you may lose your appetite.

The vagus nerve sends signals back and forth between your gut and your brain, operating in a feedback loop pattern. This can leave you with a panicky feeling. When your vagus
nerve is extremely overactivated, your blood pressure and heart rate can drop suddenly,
temporarily cutting off the blood supply to your brain. If this happens, you will feel dizzy, nau-
seated, and overheated. You could even pass out. Your "gut reaction" to stress should never be
underestimated.

Your Enteric Nervous System

When you're still in your mother's womb, some of the same nerve tissues that form your central
nervous system also form your *enteric nervous system* (*ENS*). Your ENS is comprised of approximately 100 million nerves that, among other functions, help control digestion. The vagus nerve
helps both nervous systems communicate with each other, and they use the same kinds of neurotransmitters to do so. Your enteric nervous system is housed in the walls of all 30 feet of your
gut's lining and sends signals back and forth to your brain during digestion. But the ENS does
much more than that.

Your ENS is now being termed "the second brain" by scientists who are discovering how these
bundles of nerve tissue in your gut play a role in your overall emotional and physical well-being.
The ENS doesn't do your thinking for you, but its series of neural pathways can handle the
majority of digestion independent from the brain. A growing scientific consensus in the experi-
mental fields of psychiatry and gastroenterology believe that the evolution of 100 million nerves
in the gut is too complex to deal with digestion alone.

📖 DEFINITION

> Your **vagus nerve** branches out from your brain through your chest and into your abdomen. One of its main functions is to maintain communication between your brain and digestive system. Chemicals in your nervous system that send signals between nerve cells or from your nervous system to other systems in your body are called **neurotransmitters.** The **enteric nervous system** (**ENS**) is the portion of your nervous system comprised of tens of millions of neurons and nerve cells located inside the walls of your GI tract, pancreas, and gallbladder.

Studies have shown that 90 percent of the fibers in the vagus nerve carry signals from your gut *to* your brain. Communication that one-sided surely has an impact. Your gut health and the signals the ENS sends to your brain impact your mood and play a role in disease. Serotonin is an important neurotransmitter in your body that influences mood, sexual desire, appetite, cardiovascular function, and muscle function, among other things. Most of your serotonin, 95 percent of it, is found in your gut. Most of your brain cells are influenced by serotonin, and your vagus nerve sends nearly constant signals to your brain using serotonin as one of its neurotransmitters. Additionally, 70 percent of your body's immune system is relegated to the gut.

The cutting-edge field of neurogastroenterology is studying how this mind-gut connection works. Scientists are unlocking some of the mysteries of how the gut influences the health of your immune system, mental states, and overall health. Why is this so important? Gut health is something you can gain control over. By understanding how diet and lifestyle choices affect the gut, you can empower yourself to take control of your overall well-being.

The Least You Need to Know

- Your gut's main functions are to break down food into nutrients and deliver those nutrients throughout the body.
- Your GI tract is comprised of a system of tubular organs that begin with your mouth and end with the anus.
- The trillions of bacteria that live in your gut help with digestion, nutrient absorption, and maintenance of a healthy immune system.
- Your gut and brain communicate with one another to achieve balance in your body.

CHAPTER 2

What's Normal Versus Abnormal

Most of us probably take for granted that our digestive system does all its work on autopilot. We don't pay much attention unless something is wrong. Often, however, we don't know something is abnormal until the problem is severe. There are also health issues you might not realize begin with digestive health because their symptoms materialize in places outside the gut, like the brain, joints, and the skin.

In this chapter, you learn the range considered normal for gut health. We also cover the unhealthy symptoms to watch out for and illnesses that begin in the gut.

In This Chapter

- Normal digestive states
- Normal bowel patterns
- Abnormal digestion and causes
- Common health issues that start in the gut

How to Tell If Your Gut Is Healthy

How can you tell if your gut is already pretty healthy and performing regularly? One of the most surprising ways you can keep tabs on your digestive and overall health is paying attention to the quality and frequency of your bowel movements.

That might sound uncomfortable for some of you. But this often-taboo subject is incredibly important. The shape, size, color, texture, and smell of your bowel movements can help you gauge the health of your digestive system so you can work to correct problems through diet and/ or medical intervention when necessary.

Keep in mind that there are wide ranges of normal, and you may be at one end of the spectrum or the other. It's also important to consider how you feel physically and mentally overall, what underlying discomfort or health conditions you have, and your general levels of energy.

Typical Digestion

Depending on the type of food you ate, an average meal should leave your stomach after 2 to 5 hours. That's a wide range, but meal sizes vary, and foods higher in fat take longer for the stomach to break down. Once in the small intestine, the food travels along the surface area of all those incredible villi and microvilli for several hours. The nutrients in the food residue determine the length, strength, and type of contractions your intestine generates to break down the food. Again, if the food is high in fat content, the contractions have to go on for a longer amount of time. This process can take anywhere from 3 to 10 hours.

> **GUT WISE**
>
> To improve digestion and transit time, chew your food thoroughly, eat more raw fruits and vegetables, drink at least 8 glasses of water per day *between* meals not *with* them (too much water with meals dilutes digestive juices), avoid carbonated drinks, practice portion control, add healthy fats like coconut oil and avocado, and don't exercise right after eating.

Once almost all the food residue has entered your large intestine, your small intestine will still contract in short bursts every 90 minutes in between meals or while you're sleeping to purge any "leftovers" that might linger. Once food is in your large intestine, contractions may start; this causes the rectum to stretch, giving you the urge to go. Some people's large intestine starts contracting as soon as they start eating. Everyone is different.

Normal digestion shouldn't cause pain or an uncomfortable amount of gas or bloating. Your stomach can be noisy at times, and the louder contractions that occur when you're hungry are normal. Your small intestine, large intestine, and rectum can make noise as well, but their noises should be quieter.

Bowel Movements

The fact is, your stool can tell you how well your GI tract is working as well as give you important clues about health issues outside your gut, such as neurological and autoimmune diseases. For many people, emptying their bowels is an unpleasant experience. From diarrhea to constipation, it can be pretty embarrassing. But it doesn't have to be.

About 75 percent of your stool is water. The other 25 percent is made up of old cells, mucus, fiber, and bacteria (both dead and alive). If your GI tract is working properly, and at an appropriate rate for the kinds of foods you're eating, that 25 percent should be food residue devoid of nutritional value. In other words, your bowel movements should be the garbage your body doesn't need any more. And like other garbage, it should be "taken out" often. The normal and healthy range is one to three bowel movements a day.

Consistency, size, and shape can tell you a lot about your digestive health. The ideal bowel movement is a smooth, S-shaped snake that sinks in the toilet. It should be soft and easy to pass. Sitting on the toilet should not be an event to which you take the Sunday paper or your smartphone. A few minutes is all you should need to pass a healthy, soft, stool with no pain and little effort.

Another normal side effect of the last stages of digestion is gas, or flatulence. It's healthy to pass gas. The bacteria in your large intestine release gas as they process the food residue in your gut. This gas has to go somewhere. The average person passes gas between 10 to 18 times a day.

When Is Your Gut Unhealthy?

We all experience hiccups in the regularity of a well-functioning GI tract. Most of the time these occasional deviations are nothing to be alarmed about. Overactive flatulence, bloating, heartburn, an overly noisy stomach, and bowel trouble can strike the best of us when we travel, eat exotic foods, overeat, or fall victim to minor illness. When these issues become your new norm, consult your doctor.

Other indicators of an unhealthy gut manifest outside the GI tract. Autoimmune disorders, mental-health issues, skin disorders, and vitamin deficiencies all have their root in your gut, specifically the health of your intestinal wall and the bacteria that live there.

Abnormal Digestion

One of the best gauges of whether or not you should be concerned with a digestive abnormality is recurrence. Long-term, persistent, or repeat deviations from normal digestion are cause for concern. There are likely root causes of these deviations that need to be addressed.

Bloating and gassiness happen to a lot of us during holidays, vacations, or other times of overindulgence, but these issues should not be the norm. Bloating that causes a noticeable swelling of the abdomen is often your gut's reaction to something you ate. Sometimes you bloat because you simply ate too much, but sometimes it's the kind of food that induces the gassiness. Fatty foods take longer to break down and stay in your GI tract for longer; they tend to induce that feeling of being stuffed.

> **GUT WISE**
>
> Travel-proof your digestive system to get your gut ready for your next trip. Dehydration can cause low energy, digestive issues, and cracked skin, to name a few, so carry a water bottle at all times while you're traveling. Also, move as much as possible. On road trips, stop and take a walk break, and get up once or twice on a plane to improve your circulation. Finally, bring your own food because airport, gas station, and fast food wreak havoc on your digestive system.

Sometimes bloating is caused by too much air in your GI tract. Around 50 percent of the gas in your digestive system is air you swallow. If you eat quickly, chew gum, suck on lozenges or hard candy frequently, drink carbonated beverages, or drink with a straw, you're compounding the problem. Stress and anxiety also cause people to swallow additional air. Managing stress is key to good health for myriad reasons, including reducing gas.

Some foods cause more bloating problems than others. If you eat large quantities of any of the following on a regular basis, you are contributing to bloating and uncomfortable gas: beans, lentils, Brussels sprouts, cabbage, sorbitol (an artificial sweetener), fructose, dairy products, and whole grains. Everybody's system has individual levels of tolerance for these foods. Some of them can be nutritionally dense and have valuable fiber necessary for healthy bowels, but not everyone can comfortably break down these foods, at least not in large quantities. If gas and bloating trouble you regularly, limit these foods. Drinking more water between meals can help move fiber through your GI tract and prevent bloating, too.

Abnormal bacterial overgrowth in your small intestine (sometimes referred to as small intestinal bacterial overgrowth, or SIBO) can cause severe bloating. The next time you feel so bloated you can't button your pants, and you didn't overeat or eat the healthier foods listed in the previous paragraph, take note of what comprised your last meal. Refined carbohydrates like white rice, white pasta, and white breads are especially guilty of causing SIBO and intense bloating.

Acid reflux is another reaction to specific foods. Also known as heartburn, acid reflux occurs when your stomach acid seeps into the esophagus because your lower esophageal sphincter (LES) isn't closing tightly enough. Stomach acid is strong stuff and causes a burning sensation in your upper abdomen and chest area. If this happens to you only occasionally, it isn't a major issue. But persistent, chronic heartburn can erode the lining of your esophagus and cause other serious health conditions.

Overeating, pregnancy, obesity, and constipation can contribute to acid reflux due to the increased pressure on the stomach that won't allow the lower esophageal sphincter to close properly. Some foods and substances relax the LES and promote more stomach acid production, including fatty foods, oily foods, tomatoes, citrus fruits, garlic, onion, chocolate, caffeine, and alcohol; smoking does, too. Although some of these offenders provide wonderful nutritional benefits, like citrus and garlic, if you suffer from acid reflux, limiting them might give you relief.

 YOU ARE WHAT YOU EAT

> Carbonated drinks are often consumed through straws, which adds to the air already being sent to your belly. If you are sensitive to bloating, giving up your sodas and other fizzy drinks will work wonders. In addition to water, teas are a wonderful way to increase digestion and alleviate bloating. Peppermint tea is one of the best ways to relieve bloating because it helps relax digestive muscles. (Limit peppermint if you have chronic reflux because it relaxes the LES and could worsen symptoms.)

The gurgling that occurs when gastric juices and food move through your gut are the audible sounds of the muscle contractions and sloshing within the digestive system. Sometimes, however, they can indicate something more serious. Diarrhea causes watery stools, which make louder splashing sounds as more material and gases move quickly through your gut. Occasional diarrhea is not a major problem, but chronic diarrhea can lead to dehydration, nutrient loss, and disease.

Underlying medical conditions that decrease your body's ability to break down certain foods or absorb key nutrients can also cause excessively noisy bowel sounds. If you have a problem digesting substances that reach the large intestine unabsorbed and undigested, the bacteria in your gut will cause those substances to ferment and release gas, create more fluid, and stimulate contractions. Gas, fluid, and contractions are the three conditions necessary for abdominal noise.

Some people experience exaggerated digestive sounds accompanied by intense pain and lethargy. These could indicate a medical emergency—the intestinal pathway might be dangerously narrow, and contractions might be trying to force the liquid, gas, and solids through an insufficient opening. On the other hand, if your bowels are making *no* noise at all and you experience intense abdominal pain, there is also a likelihood of a medical emergency. If your GI noise is out of the ordinary or disrupts your quality of life, seek professional medical advice.

Bowel troubles are often the most undiagnosed of problems because people let their embarrassment prevent them from talking openly about them, even with their doctors. Remember, the material expelled by your anus is waste. It contains toxins that need to be eliminated. If you're not having at least one bowel movement a day on a regular basis, there may be a problem. Temporary irregularity from travel or sickness is an exception. It's long-term deviation from the one to three daily bowel movements that should cause concern.

If you only poop a couple times a week, you're most likely constipated and need to drink more water between meals and slowly increase your fiber intake. If you are going more than five times a day and your stools are watery or loose, you're suffering from chronic diarrhea. Both ends of the spectrum can cause irritation in your gut, which can contribute to serious health issues.

Constipation is also a problem because it causes you to have to push harder when evacuating your bowels. This strains your rectal tissues and can cause tears, bleeding, and enlarged blood vessels called *hemorrhoids*. Irritation of the colorectal tissues make future bowel movements uncomfortable and even difficult. And constipation can lead to a feeling that you always have some fecal material left behind, which might indicate that your bowel movements really aren't complete.

In addition to frequency and ease of evacuation, check the quality of the stools themselves. If they float, they probably have too much fat in them, which could indicate your small intestine is having problems absorbing fats and potentially other nutrients. Your doctor and dietitian can perform tests to see if you have a gluten intolerance or if your pancreas is inflamed. Pencil-thin bowel movements are often caused by diarrhea, but persistent thin stools are sometimes the result of *colorectal polyps* or cancer.

> **DEFINITION**
>
> When tissues in the colorectal area become inflamed, they lead to enlarged blood vessels called **hemorrhoids. Colorectal polyps** are growths that extend outward from colon and rectum tissues. Sometimes they're harmless, but they can be cancerous and should be evaluated and/or removed by a doctor.

Healthy stool should be shades of brown or green. Unusual-colored stools like bright red, white, light clay, or black are cause for concern. Sometimes beets can make your stool bright red, but so can bleeding near the end of the digestive tract. Certain medications can turn your poop white, but so can a lack of bile, an important digestive fluid. Licorice can turn your stools black, but so can stomach bleeding. It's always best to have something that is out of the ordinary checked by a doctor.

Another indicator that bowel movements are unhealthy is a fouler than normal smell, which can indicate the presence of an intestinal parasite. Persistent pungency could be a sign of ulcerative colitis, Crohn's disease, or celiac disease. Again, try to get past your initial embarrassment and talk to a health-care professional if these abnormalities persist.

Mental-Health Issues

In addition to the physical symptoms of gut problems, also take stock of your mental well-being. Knowing how the brain and gut interact, it should be no surprise that psychological states impact gut function and vice versa. Stress, anxiety, lack of focus, and other mental issues can all be linked to an unhealthy gut.

When you're feeling stressed out or depressed, your brain sends signals throughout your body, including your GI tract. Stress can affect the kinds of contractions and gastric juices released in the gut; this can cause nausea, intestinal pain, and even inflammation, which leaves you vulnerable to infection. All the symptoms of abnormal digestion we've discussed (acid reflux, abnormal bowel movements, excessive gas, and bloating) can be caused or exacerbated by stress.

Poor nutrition, contributing to overpopulation of bad bacteria in the gut, can also lead to mental symptoms or could make preexisting mental symptoms worse. Your enteric nervous system might send signals back to your brain that can disrupt hormone levels, lead to anxiety, and contribute to an increase in the perception of stress and feelings of depression.

GUT WISE

If you experience a combination of muscle tension (especially neck and shoulders); problems sleeping; teeth grinding; social withdrawal; and/or anxiety, depression, and lack of focus, you may be experiencing mental issues whose root causes lie in the gut.

Reducing stress through meditative exercises, therapy, and exercise can actually improve GI function and alleviate negative symptoms. Likewise, making lifestyle and nutrition choices that foster optimal gut health can lessen the severity of stress, anxiety, and even more serious mood disorders. (We discuss more specific impacts of gut health on mental well-being in Chapter 7.)

Vitamin Deficiencies

Your small intestine is divided into three parts that each break down and absorb different key nutrients essential to overall health. The duodenum digests fats and fat-soluble vitamins like A, D, E, and K. The jejunum performs about 90 percent of your nutrient absorption, which consists of proteins, water soluble vitamins, carbohydrates, and minerals. The ileum absorbs water, bile salts, and vitamin B_{12}. A healthy small intestine works hard to absorb nutrients. If your small intestine is not absorbing nutrients properly, it can lead to vitamin deficiencies that impair normal growth and development, digestive and nervous system functions, and mental capacity.

Calcium and vitamin D are often discussed together because they affect bone health and work best in the body when ingested simultaneously. Calcium helps maintain bone health and strength and muscle and nerve function. If you're low on calcium, you might just feel tired and lose your appetite, or you might experience more extreme symptoms like muscle cramps or an abnormal heartbeat.

When most people think of healthy sources of calcium they automatically think "milk." This response is largely the result of very successful dairy-industry campaigns. Later in this book, we discuss healthy dairy options for those who can tolerate dairy, but there are lots of foods that have just as much calcium as milk and milk products. For example, ½ cup tofu; 10 dried figs; and 3 ounces salmon, sardines, or mackerel have just as much calcium as an 8-ounce glass of milk. Other foods rich in calcium include white beans, black-eyed peas, almonds, sesame seeds, bok choy, kale, turnip greens, seaweed, blackstrap molasses, and oranges.

Vitamin D deficiency has increased dramatically over the past 20 years. According to the Centers for Disease Control and Prevention (CDC), in the United States alone, at least 25 percent of the population is deficient. That's alarming considering the important role vitamin D plays. It's responsible for maintaining the health of bones, muscle, the heart, and the immune system (70 percent of which is concentrated in your gut). Science is now linking a lack of vitamin D to diseases like diabetes and cancer.

Symptoms of vitamin D deficiency include fatigue, an increase in the number and severity of infections (like the common cold), muscle pain and weakness, bone pain, and softening of the bones. One of the best ways to get more vitamin D is to expose yourself to direct sunlight without sunscreen. In light of skin cancer concerns, this isn't happening as much for some people as it used to. The key here is to exercise moderation and caution. If you're fair-skinned, you only need about 15 minutes of direct exposure when the sun is at its highest point in the sky. If you're dark-skinned, you will need longer, up to 2 hours. Estimate what you need by exposing yourself for half the time it would normally take you to burn. You want the benefits of vitamin D without risking sunburn. If this is a balancing act you don't feel comfortable with, vitamin D–fortified foods and supplements are available.

GUT WISE

New research shows a correlation between muscle function and vitamin D. Yet another reason to take a walk in the sunshine and absorb what you need while improving your overall health. And while you're outside, don't be afraid to get a little dirty as well. Beneficial bacteria in the soil can actually help your digestive system!

Potassium depletion is very common in people with unhealthy guts. Potassium enables some major organs to function properly, like the kidneys and heart. Potassium is mostly absorbed by the first section of your large intestine. This is one of the reasons why you can become depleted in the short term if you suffer from diarrhea. Vomiting and excessive sweating also contribute to short-term potassium depletion.

Long-term potassium deficiencies can occur due to kidney disease or irritable bowels that cause chronic diarrhea. Symptoms of potassium depletion include weight loss, muscle weakness, constipation, and even an irregular heartbeat. Bananas are a well-known potassium source, but so are sweet potatoes, kale, peas, and Swiss chard.

Poor gut health can also impede iron absorption. Without enough iron, your body can't make enough red blood cells to effectively carry oxygen throughout the body. This condition is called *anemia*. Anemia will leave you feeling drained and lethargic. It can also cause pale skin and thinning, dull hair. Supplements are often necessary to combat anemia, but some foods that can naturally boost iron levels are beef, oysters, beans, lentils, and spinach.

Vitamin B_{12} is absorbed in the ileum of your small intestine and your large intestine. It helps with DNA productions and brain neurotransmitters. If you're low in this vitamin, you may experience numbness in your extremities, dizziness that leads to balance problems, anemia, fatigue, an irritated or swollen tongue, memory problems, confusion, and even hallucinations. Vitamin B_{12} is only found in animal products and supplements. You can boost your B_{12} levels naturally with foods like eggs, fish, beef, and yogurt.

DEFINITION

> **Anemia** occurs when the ability of the blood to deliver oxygen to body systems has been compromised due to low iron and vitamin B_{12} levels.

Magnesium deficiency is one of the more uncommon deficiencies. However, if your gut is out of whack, or you have other underlying health conditions that require you to take medication, or if you drink a lot of alcohol, you can fall victim to a magnesium deficiency. Magnesium helps with bone health and energy levels. If you're low in this mineral, you'll experience fatigue, weakness, nausea, and even vomiting. Extremely low levels can cause numbness, cramps, seizures, abnormal heartbeat, and contribute to even lower potassium and calcium levels. You can increase your levels naturally with almonds, cashews, spinach, black beans, and soy beans.

Vitamin deficiencies are problems that usually begin in the gut and are directly related to the health of the gut microbes (see Chapter 3). If you're not absorbing vital nutrients, then they can't be delivered to the rest of your body systems. The symptoms covered in this section can help you troubleshoot whether or not your intestine is healthy enough to perform this task optimally.

If you experience any or all of these symptoms, ask your health-care provider for blood tests to confirm vitamin depletion and to rule out other health issues.

Some symptoms of vitamin deficiency are similar to those of other illnesses, and some of the symptoms are rather vague (like fatigue). If a doctor or dietitian concludes you have a vitamin deficiency, the good news is it can be remediated through diet. Some doctors and dietitians will suggest supplements, but these should only be necessary in the short term. Eating a diet that is nutrient-rich will alleviate vitamin deficiencies and lead to a healthy gut.

Antibiotic Use

Anyone who's had a raging infection of some kind understands that antibiotics can literally be a lifesaver. But consider the meaning of the word itself. *Antibiotic* means "against life." They are wonder drugs designed to kill bacteria that cause disease. The downside to this miracle medicine is that it also kills some of the good bacteria that live in the gut.

As we discuss in more detail in Chapter 3, your GI tract is host to trillions of bacteria that aid in digestion, immunity, and gut-brain communication. The relationship our body has with these organisms is just starting to be more fully understood by scientists, and the health implications are manifold. One thing is certain when it comes to gut bacteria, antibiotics disrupt the balance.

Beneficial gut bacteria die-off is a major side effect of antibiotic use that doesn't get enough attention. Often the harmful bacteria repopulate your gut before the good bacteria have a chance to catch up. This imbalance can change the way your gut bacteria communicates with the lining of your intestine, throwing off the entire process of nutrient absorption and transport to the other body systems. The end results of gut bacteria imbalance can lead to digestive discomfort, irritable bowel syndrome (IBS), yeast infections, and even mental issues.

> **GUT WISE**
>
> Although antibiotics are sometimes necessary, they are certainly overprescribed in the United States. A whopping four out of five people are prescribed a course every year. Discuss the risks and benefits of antibiotics thoroughly with your doctor before you go to the pharmacy.

If you've used antibiotics at some point in the past, and most of us have, there is a strong likelihood you've disrupted the balance of bacteria in your gut. And it may have compromised your GI tract's ability to run at optimal levels. How do we balance our digestive needs with our need to recover from often serious infections?

While you're on antibiotics, and immediately after finishing a course of antibiotics, avoid sugar and simple carbohydrates. Simple carbohydrates are converted very quickly into sugars by the body. Avoiding these foods is helpful in achieving a healthy gut in general, but it's especially important while your body is recovering from illness and the ravaging of good bacteria. Pathogenic bacteria thrive on sugar. If you avoid sugar and simple carbohydrates, you starve your gut's enemy.

Simple Versus Complex Carbs

Carb Type	Sugar Composition	Digestion Impact	Nutrient Density	Examples
Simple carbs	One or two sugar molecules	Rapidly converted into sugar	Low in nutrients	Table sugar, corn syrup, fruit drinks, soda, candy, honey, jams, molasses, white breads, pastas, and rice
Complex carbs	String of complex sugar molecules	Slowly digested, often combined with fiber and makes you feel full	Nutrient rich	Green vegetables, oatmeal, whole-grain pastas and breads, sweet potatoes, squash, beans, pea, and lentils

Promoting the repopulation of good bacteria is not just about starving the bad, it's also about actively replenishing healthy gut bacteria. Ingesting foods that are *probiotics* can help. Fermented and cultures foods (like yogurt, tempeh, kefir, kimchi, pickles, and raw sauerkraut) contain live bacteria that can assist in repopulating your gut. (We talk more about cultured and fermented foods in Chapter 11 and how to make your own in Chapter 14.) Taking a store-bought probiotic in pill, liquid, or powdered form can be effective but also expensive.

Food Sensitivities and Allergies

While the exact causes of food allergies are still somewhat of an enigma, today's scientists are finding the answers lie in our gut. If you suffer from food sensitivities or food allergies, it may be another sign that your GI tract is not functioning properly, specifically, that your gut bacteria are not in balance. If you don't replenish the good bacteria after a round of antibiotics, there can be long-term effects, like food allergies.

Many factors put our GI tracts at risk for developing food allergies. Some studies suggest the modern diet and overuse of antibacterial cleaning and personal hygiene products contribute to the problem. Some of our daily practices strip our systems of the helpful bacteria that would prevent our bodies from having adverse reactions to foods.

Scientific studies at the University of Chicago in 2014 have isolated one strain of bacteria in particular, *clostridia,* for its role in protecting us from food allergies. What makes Clostridia special is its ability to communicate with immune cells in the gut, signaling them to produce a molecule that prevents holes in the lining of your intestine. Clostridia can actually reduce the symptoms of a leaky gut.

> **DEFINITION**
>
> **Probiotics** are beneficial bacteria and are crucial to our digestive health. Some strains of bacteria, like **clostridia,** have both harmful and helpful varieties. Some clostridia strains cause deadly infections like tetanus, while other protect us from developing food allergies.

Fewer undigested food particles and pathogens in your bloodstream means your immune system won't overreact to them with the inflammatory responses we know as food allergies. But if your gut bacteria are not diverse and in balance, then chances are your population of clostridia bacteria might not be strong enough to help ward off food allergies.

If you have severe allergies, you probably already know it. Severe allergic reactions to food can be life-threatening. Your body might go into shock, or your lips, tongue, or throat might swell. Some people have difficulty swallowing or breathing; this could even lead to a loss of consciousness.

More mild allergic reactions to food sometimes manifest as chronic but manageable conditions that people become used to treating with prescription or over-the-counter drugs. They might not even be aware that these conditions are actually allergic reactions to food that begin in the gut. These chronic conditions are the skin and autoimmune conditions we discuss next.

Skin Issues and Disorders

The idea that gut health might be connected to skin health goes back to research conducted as early as 1916. More recent studies worldwide have confirmed the links. People with severe gastrointestinal disorders like ulcerative colitis, celiac disease, and Crohn's often have skin problems as well. And the link can be followed in the opposite direction; people who suffer from severe acne are 10 times more likely to have small intestinal bacterial overgrowth (SIBO) that disrupts gut function. They are also more likely to have intestinal hyperpermeability ("leaky gut"), which leeches more harmful bacteria into the body's systems, causing inflammation in other places like the skin.

Gut inflammation can negatively influence the skin's ability to serve as a protective barrier for the entire body. When the skin's integrity is compromised, it's left vulnerable to infection and inflammation. Probiotics can help alleviate skin disorders like eczema, acne, seborrheic dermatitis, and psoriasis. Heal the gut and inflammation elsewhere in the body will be healed as well—even on your skin.

Autoimmune Disorders and Diseases

New research confirms that most *autoimmune disorders* begin in the gut, specifically in the lining of the intestine. Statistics on the rise of autoimmune disease are disheartening, with nearly 50 million Americans alone affected by the disorders.

Autoimmune disease occurs when the immune system is overstimulated and your body's natural defenses mistakenly attack your body's healthy tissues. These illnesses can occur in any of your body's systems. Because most of your body's immune cells, your enteric nervous system, and the main nutrient transport systems to the rest of your body, reside in the small intestine, it is only logical to conclude that autoimmune illness starts in the gut.

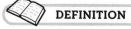 **DEFINITION**

> **Autoimmune disorders** are a category of diseases that cause a person's immune system to attack his or her own healthy cells and tissues.

The following are some of the most common autoimmune diseases and their symptoms:

- **Rheumatoid arthritis:** Swollen painful joints
- **Lupus:** Inflammation of skin and joints, systemic problems with organs such as the brain and kidneys
- **Multiple sclerosis:** Inflammation in the brain and spinal cord
- **Celiac disease:** Inflammation of the small intestinal lining in reaction to gluten
- **Anemia:** Decrease in red blood cells due to compromised ability to absorb vitamin B_{12}
- **Psoriasis:** Inflammation and redness of the skin often in thick, flaky patches

- **Inflammatory bowel disease (IBD, including IBS and Crohn's):** Inflammation of small intestine and colon

- **Hashimoto's disease:** Inflammation of thyroid

- **Type 1 diabetes:** Pancreatic cell destruction

If you have any of these diseases, or any of the other nearly 80 identified categories of auto-immune diseases, chances are you have bacterial overgrowth or imbalance in the gut, which interferes with its important functions. According to many doctors and scientists (and to the prominent Dr. Alessio Fasano, whose research is discussed in more depth in Chapter 5), three major factors form the root of all autoimmune disease:

- A person already has the genes for the disease

- A person has been exposed to antigens (which are allergens or irritants that cause a reaction)

- A person has increased intestinal permeability ("leaky gut")

In short, if you already have the genes for an autoimmune disorder, and your gut and its bacteria aren't balanced and functioning properly, then harmful antigens and undigested food can be circulated throughout your body, causing your immune system to attack healthy tissues. The silver lining, however, is that many symptoms of autoimmune disease, even in severe cases, can be mitigated or even reversed through diet.

The Least You Need to Know

- Normal digestion should be painless and comfortable.
- Unhealthy gut signs include excessive bloating and gas, and irregular bowel movements.
- Underlying conditions that start in the gut include mental-health issues, skin problems, autoimmune disease, and vitamin deficiencies.
- Genetics, increased intestinal permeability, and gut-bacteria imbalance can lead to disease.
- Diet and lifestyle choices can help heal your gut by restoring balance to gut bacteria and repairing intestinal hyperpermeability.

Microflora and the Autoimmune Balancing Act

As kids, we learned about ecosystems primarily on a large scale. An ecosystem is a group of organisms, large and small, interacting with each other within a specific environment. Forests, deserts, and grasslands are all examples of large ecosystems. You probably took a test somewhere along the line where you defined *ecosystem* alongside terms like *species* and *habitat*. This working vocabulary helps us understand the checks and balances among life on this planet. But do we ever really think of the ecosystems that live *inside* of us?

In this chapter, you learn there is virtually another planet's worth of ecosystems living inside of you right now; how the microscopic ecosystems of the human body are vulnerable to disruption and imbalance; and if we can understand how our personal "gut ecosystems" work and keep them balanced, we can optimize our chances for excellent health.

In This Chapter

- Microflora, a vital part of our internal ecosystem
- The importance of the brain-gut axis
- Causes of microflora imbalances
- The role of "tight junctions" in managing intestinal health
- A healthy immune system begins in the gut

Microflora: The Ecosystem in Your Gut

In your body at this very minute are trillions, yes trillions, of tiny organisms called *microbes* that help your body function properly. Instead of getting squirmy, try to appreciate them for all the work they do. They communicate with our nervous, immune, and circulatory systems. Without the enzymes they produce, there are many nutrients we would be unable to absorb on our own.

Throughout the history of humankind these bacteria have evolved alongside us. Collectively, all the microbes living in and on our bodies is called the human *microbiome*. It may seem gross to think of ourselves as the habitat for tiny organisms, but these organisms help us stay healthy.

What Is Microflora?

The world is full of bacteria, algae, and fungi, and we are the hosts for a lot of them. *Microflora* is the term given to describe a collection of these types of organisms that live together in a certain habitat. The microflora that live in the digestive tracts of animals and humans are sometimes called "gut flora" or *microbiota*. We have a lot of tiny organisms that use our bodies as their habitat, but the microflora in our digestive system is the largest population of them all.

> **DEFINITION**
>
> **Microbes** are tiny bacteria, both beneficial and harmful. The collection of microbes that live together in a particular environment is called a **microbiome. Microbiota** is the more accepted and common term for "gut flora" or **microflora,** which are the microbes that live in the digestive tracts of animals and humans.

Tens of trillions of microorganisms live in your digestive tract. Your intestines are home to about 1,000 different species of bacteria. If we gathered up the entire population of microbiota in your body, they would weigh between 2 and 3 pounds. The microbial cells in our body outnumber human cells 10 to 1. Microbiota are also more genetically complex than a human being. They have 150 times more genes than we do.

Your individual combination of microbiota is unlike anyone else's. Sure, there are some species that most people have. Roughly one third of your gut microbes are just like everyone else's. But the other two thirds? That's all you. Our population of microbiota are like snowflakes—no two people are exactly alike. Your gut flora is as unique as your fingerprint.

We should be very curious about these microorganisms who call us home and work to keep them happy and working in harmony with our bodies' systems. There are many reasons why we should pay attention to our relationship with these organisms. Gut bacteria evolved alongside humans to work symbiotically with our bodies.

What Do Microbiota Do?

Even though everyone's exact population makeup of microbiota is different, the jobs of that population are the same. One of the main functions of the microbiota is to aid in the digestion of foods that aren't completely digested in the stomach and small intestine. They also regulate the wholeness of the mucus that lines the tubes of the intestinal wall. This gut mucosa protects the intestines from invading microorganisms that don't belong in the gut.

The microbiota are like the bodyguards of your intestine, saying, "Get out!" to invaders that will only wreak havoc if they get into your digestive tract. Bacteria from your own gut basically compete for nutrition sources in your intestine and for attachments sites on the intestinal wall. The more of these healthy bacteria you have growing, the less susceptible you are to having harmful microbes gaining too much territory in your gut.

Healthy gut bacteria thrive on dietary fiber. If your starve them of their food source they eat … us. This sounds like creepy science fiction, but it's true. Bad bacteria will eat the mucus lining in your large intestine, which over time could damage its ability to function properly. Just another reason to feed these populations the right kinds of foods.

 YOU ARE WHAT YOU EAT

Eat more garlic and leeks! Not only are they delicious, but they contain a powerful prebiotic called inulin. A prebiotic is a substance that promotes the growth of good probiotic bacteria in your gut.

Science is learning how this population of organisms contribute to the effectiveness of our immune system by actually communicating with our digestive and nervous systems. The microbiota also help make two important vitamins: B vitamins, which help our energy levels and red blood cell development; and vitamin K, which helps the body create proteins necessary to clot blood and maintain bone health. This tiny ecosystem living in your gut plays a major role in your overall health.

Where Do We Get Our Microbiota?

In short, your mom gives them to you. When babies pass through the vaginal canal at birth, they pick up all kinds of microbial gifts from their moms along the way. A baby's microbial community is populated by hitchhikers from the mom's system. A baby born via cesarean section picks up her microbes primarily from her mother's and father's skin.

Babies also inherit their microbiota from their mother's breast milk. When a complex carbohydrate that infants don't have the ability to digest was discovered in breast milk, scientists were left scratching their heads. Why on earth would evolution allow for this seemingly useless carbohydrate to exist in breast milk?

After further study, scientists concluded that the carbohydrate was there not to feed the baby, but to feed a special microbe in the baby's gut that nourishes the lining of the intestines, protecting it from inflammation and infection. The makers of infant formula now take this into consideration and include man-made complex carbohydrates in their products that support a community of microbiota similar to breast-fed babies.

> **GUT WISE**
>
> While breastfeeding is an intensely personal choice, if you're healthy and capable, breastfeeding is the best way to ensure your baby has the best shot at a healthy immune system. Human breast milk contains carbohydrates that interact with a bacteria called *Bifidobacterium longum infantis*. The carbohydrates "teach" those specific bacteria found only in infants how to respond to pathogens. It teaches the bacteria how to be bodyguards. It remains uncertain whether the man-made carbohydrates in formula can ever perform this same task.

The Microbiome and Your Brain

In Chapter 2, we learned how the trillions of bacteria living in your gut communicate with your brain via the vagus nerve pathway. This "conversation" is often referred to as the brain-gut axis. Science is uncovering the relationship between your gut and your mental well-being, and your microbiota play a huge role in this.

The Vagus Nerve and Bacteria Imbalance

The vagus nerve is a busy communication highway between your gut and brain. Bacterial imbalance in the gut affects brain activity and function and vice versa. Decreased activity in the brain decreases activity in the vagus nerve. The vagus nerve activates gut motility, and gets your GI tract moving and secreting necessary juices. If it's not communicating signals properly, the result might be a decrease in blood flow to the intestine and compromised intestinal immune function.

Poor intestinal immunity causes an overgrowth of pathogenic bacteria and yeasts. This major disruption in the microbiota can lead to increased intestinal permeability. A leaky gut promotes inflammation, which can pose serious health risks.

GUT WISE

In a 2014 scientific report published by the National Institutes of Health (NIH), mice were given traumatic brain injuries that caused damage to the vagus nerve. With the integrity of their communication highway for the brain-gut axis destroyed, the mice developed increased intestinal permeability (leaky gut syndrome) in just 6 hours!

Leaky Gut, Leaky Brain: A Vicious Cycle

If the gut is out of whack, specialized immune cells produce *cytokines*, which are molecules that send signals to other immune cells communicating it's time to induce an inflammatory response. Inflammatory immune cells then travel through the blood, crossing the blood-brain barrier causing further inflammation in the brain. Overactive intestinal permeability and the havoc it wreaks on microbiota balance lead to poor immune function and inflammation in the brain. This cycle worsens as brain inflammation continues to weaken the brain-gut axis, which results in even more inflammatory cytokines flowing to the brain.

This negative cycle of inflammation can even lead to depression. It also leads to more gut agitation because the signals being sent for digestive function are compromised. Anxiety, stress, irritable bowel syndrome (IBS) and irritable bowel disease (IBD, like ulcerative colitis and Crohn's disease) are all connected. Every stressful experience we have increases the brain's ability to run stress pathways more efficiently. More stress means crossed signals, microbiota imbalance, and impaired gut function.

GUT WISE

Symptoms of brain-gut axis problems include brain fog, fatigue, chronic digestive issues, anxiety, depression, autism spectrum disorders, behavioral problems, cold hands and feet, and toenail fungus.

How We Damage Our Tiny Ecosystems

In today's world, it's all too easy to engage in behavior that disturbs the balance of our intestinal terrain. Let's break down these eight major culprits and explain how each of them adversely affect your gut.

Genetics: Unfortunately, some people are genetically predisposed to digestive problems and may have inherited poor-quality microbiota.

Prolonged use of antibiotics (at any age): Antibiotics are often life-saving. But be wary of using them for minor illnesses. Anytime antibiotics are used, they kill off a lot of the good bacteria in the gut along with the bad. They run through your digestive tract like a natural disaster, and it takes time for that microflora to get reestablished. Sometimes, the good bacteria never recover.

Travel (especially outside of one's native country): When we travel, we are exposed to new bacteria. When our body is introduced to something foreign, it can often cause an imbalance.

Poor diet: Poor nutrition will promote the growth of the worst kinds of bacteria and yeasts in your gut. This can lead to digestive discomfort, and, in extreme cases, digestive diseases.

Stress: Too much stress isn't good for any of your body's systems. Your digestive tract and its inhabitants are no exception.

Food intolerance: Some people might not have full-blown allergic reactions to certain foods, but their bodies might still have difficulty processing them. These intolerances can damage the balance of good flora in the gut and compromise the lining of the intestine. Likewise, the microbiota can actually cause the food intolerance. This "culprit" is a two-way street.

Leaky gut syndrome: If your microbiota have been out of whack for a long time, your intestinal wall might be damaged, allowing undigested food particles into the bloodstream and harmful bacteria into your digestive tract. Without healing the gut, this can be a never-ending vicious cycle.

Nature deprivation: Numerous scientific studies demonstrate that a primarily "indoors" existence can deprive you of exposure to good bacteria. Getting your hands dirty in soil by gardening, taking deep breaths in fresh air outdoors, these activities increase the diversity of your microbiota. You'll be less likely to have allergies and more likely to be healthy.

The good news about all of these culprits is that they can be managed. You can't change your genetics, but you can manage your microbiota population to ensure that only the best kinds of bacteria are growing. You can control your use of antibiotics and eat food rich in natural probiotics or take probiotics supplements to help encourage the growth of healthy microbiota when you're traveling and when you're enduring periods of high stress. You can make an effort to spend more time outdoors.

You can also learn to recognize your body's reactions to foods that make you feel bloated or that trigger adverse reactions anywhere in your body. (For more details on these reactions see the "When Is Your Gut Unhealthy" section in Chapter 2.)

YOU ARE WHAT YOU EAT

The soluble fiber in chia seeds allows them to swell up and create a gel by pulling in water which promotes overall gut health, feeds your gut flora, and helps to stabilize blood sugar. Chia seeds stimulate your small intestine much like a brush or a broom, which is important for digestion to help keep things moving along to the large intestine. Chia seeds can be used in jams, puddings, smoothies, and in baking as a thickener. They are a great topping for yogurt, fruit, and oatmeal.

"Tight Junctions" and Your Intestinal Health

Our bodies have built-in protective mechanisms to protect against invaders while allowing the good stuff to pass. Your mouth doesn't remain open all the time and neither do the openings in your intestinal wall. There are tiny spaces between each of the cells that line your gut. These spaces have gatekeepers called tight junctions that work like swinging doors. They're flexible structures that, in healthy individuals, only open wide enough for nutrients to pass into the circulatory system.

Tight junctions play a critical role in the health of your intestine. They work with your gut bacteria to make sure you're absorbing nutrients and fighting off bad pathogens. In order for everything to run smoothly in your gut, tight junctions have to be healthy and so does your microbiome.

What Are Tight Junctions?

Epithelial cells are the types of cells that line the surfaces of structures in our body like our skin, the lining of our stomach, and the lining of our intestines. Inside these cells are specialized structures called tight junctions that are kind of spot-welded to the *plasma membrane* of the cells. They almost look like stitches that "tape" the cells of your intestinal wall, enterocytes, together.

When unhealthy microbiota imbalances cause tight junction malfunction, these cellular gate-keepers open too widely and cause what is often referred to as "leaky gut syndrome." When the spaces between the enterocytes in your gut lining get too wide, a whole host of problems can arise.

> **DEFINITION**
>
> **Cytokines** are molecules that help with cell to cell communication and stimulate the movement of white blood cells to the sites of infection, damage, and inflammation in the body. Cells that make up the thin surface layer of body structures, especially tubular structures like those in our GI tracts are called **epithelial cells.** A **plasma membrane** is the boundary of a cell's internal material that controls the passage of foreign matter in and out of the cell.

Tight Junctions and Your Microbiota

Tight junctions are constantly reacting to outside stimuli. They change their structure according to their interactions with the microbiota in your intestines. They're basically like highly impressionable teenagers. So you want to make sure the microbiota they come into contact with are healthy—you know, "the good kids." The quality of their interactions with microbiota affect the way tight junctions perform their jobs of regulating the entry of nutrients and water into the intestine and keeping nasty stuff like pathogens out.

When your microbiota are out of whack, your enterocytes aren't at optimal health. Any of the eight major culprits mentioned earlier in this chapter can cause a microbiota imbalance that can ultimately cause your tight junctions to come "unglued." Tight junctions that stay open too long leave wide gaps between enterocytes. If these gaps are plentiful and extreme, a leaky gut ensues.

These holes in the intestinal walls let undigested particles of food into surrounding tissues, which in turn cause some people's immune systems to go into overdrive. People with food intolerances, especially to gluten or dairy, or who have genetic predispositions to immune diseases, are especially at risk for these types of responses. The immune system registers these food particles as foreign invaders and then mistakenly starts attacking healthy tissues in the body. These attacks are the root of a whole range of nasty health problems.

Immunity Begins in the Gut

Between 70 and 80 percent of your immune tissue is in your GI tract. The microbes that live in your gut play a role in the effectiveness of your immune response to pathogens who find their way into your digestive system. The strains of beneficial bacteria in your intestines work in conjunction with your immune cells to help them achieve maximum infection-fighting capacity. How they do this is a fascinating study in symbiosis.

Microbes: The Protectors Against Pathogens

Gut bacteria have the ability to produce substances that are harmful to the pathogenic bacteria and send signals to the gut mucosa to produce compounds that are antimicrobial; it's like your own internal soap that kills germs. Your gut produces immune cells, hormones, and various signaling substances important to bodily functions. One of its molecular messenger substances, antimicrobial peptides (AMPs), helps protect you from pathogenic bacteria. AMPs have the capacity to change the surface structure of bacteria, so they can't properly function. They're like discreet bouncers who get rid of obnoxious party guests. Microbiologists are discovering that these substances seem to be produced strategically so that they alter the populations of bacteria in a way that benefits us, their host.

One of the main functions of the molecular messenger substances created in the gut is to control which bacteria make up the intestinal microbiota population and how many of each kind of bacteria will thrive. These substances interact with the microbiota. There are even microbiota that encourage you, the host, to make even more messenger molecules. The exact mechanisms at work in these interactions aren't fully known, but emerging science shows the result of these interactions is the regulation of healthy gut bacteria populations.

GUT WISE

Beneficial bacteria not only help with your immune system and digestion, but emerging science suggests they might even absorb harmful cancer-causing substances that make their way into the body.

Keeping the Intestinal Barrier Intact

The gastrointestinal immune cells secrete white blood cells that attack pathogens. These white blood cells also bundle together to form structures known as Peyer's patches on the mucous membranes on the last section of the small-intestinal wall. These patches release specialized white blood cells (called T-cells and B-cells) that work together to protect the intestinal barrier from infection and damage.

The Peyer's patches communicate with the microbes in your gut to determine if they're healthy or they pose a threat. This helps regulate healthy microbial populations in your gut and prevents pathogens from growing unchecked. The Peyer's patches send signals to the lymphatic system to boost your whole body's immune response and make sure infectious threats don't travel beyond the intestines. It's another mechanism that operates like that helpful nightclub bouncer.

The checks and balances in a healthy functioning gut will promote the growth of certain probiotic bacteria. These probiotics protect you from pathogens by preventing invasive species from attaching to your intestinal wall. And your intestinal wall needs these microbes. In fact, the epithelial cells of the gut get 60 to 70 percent of their energy from the activity of bacteria. You want that energy to be positive. Additionally, gut bacteria help maintain the healthy production of enterocytes. If the makeup of our gut bacteria is imbalanced, the intestinal lining doesn't receive proper nourishment or cell renewal, setting the stage for a damaged gut wall that can't properly absorb nutrients and keep tight junctions healthy.

Probiotic bacteria basically launch attacks against pathogenic bacteria. Scientists are still examining exactly how and why these crafty bacteria act this way, but the end result is often protection of the host from infection. And since we're their host, we should celebrate their tactics and do whatever we can to promote their healthy presence in our gut.

Lactobacillus and *Bifidobacterium* (two probiotic strains commonly found in cultured dairy products) are very good at protecting our intestinal barrier. These good bacteria secrete compounds that activate the immune response in the cells of your intestinal wall to fight off pathogens (specifically listeria and E. coli). *Lactobacillus* specifically also produces lactic acid. This is great news for our guts because a lot of pathogenic bacteria can't grow in the presence of lactic acid. Additionally, lactic acid causes our gut lining to produce natural microbial enzymes that disrupt the membranes of nasty bacteria. The internal soap that kills germs strikes again!

Achieving Gut Homeostasis

Symbiosis is a state of mutual benefit. In our gut, mechanisms are at work to sustain the symbiosis between our microbiota and the smooth sailing of other body systems. When everything is functioning optimally, we are in a state of *homeostasis*. Homeostasis is the ultimate goal of biological function; it's when everything is in perfect balance.

In order to achieve this balance in the gut, the healthy bacteria have to crowd out the pathogenic ones. We can help the bacteria with these jobs by trying not to overtax our system with toxins and foods that trigger negative responses in our body and feed the populations of harmful bacteria.

> **DEFINITION**
>
> **Homeostasis** is a state of equilibrium or balance; it's what all biological systems strive to achieve.

Healthy Bacteria Crowd Out Pathogens

Your gut microbiota are your first line of defense against invading pathogens that come in contact with your GI tract. One of the ways they provide protection is to simply crowd out the invaders. They occupy attachment sites on the lining of the intestinal wall so others can't get there. They consume nutrient sources first before the nasty bacteria have a chance. These combined strategies are called competitive exclusion. It's a "safety in numbers" tactic.

Healthy bacteria, and the by-products of their metabolism (which is their consumption of nutrients and then giving off waste products), can stimulate your gut to produce AMPs, those awesome molecular messenger substances that will disrupt the surface structures of bacteria. This defense simultaneously helps protect you against invading pathogens and prevents too many of one species of indigenous bacteria from overcrowding your gut. If homeostasis is disrupted, meticulous attention to diet and eliminating toxins is the only way to reestablish the beneficial bacteria that make symbiosis possible.

Gut Homeostasis Keeps Candida in Check

In addition to bacteria, your gut is host to other microbes like a fungus called candida. Candida is symbiotic with its host if its population is kept in check. Candida even helps with digestion and nutrient absorption. Unfortunately, it's one of the most common overgrowth problems in the human gut. A population boom of candida can cause damage in the intestinal lining and contribute to leaky gut.

Symptoms of candida overgrowth are similar to those of small intestinal bacterial overgrowth (SIBO), brain-gut axis problems, and leaky gut in general. These symptoms all overlap because their underlying root cause is a disruption in healthy gut microbiota, which make gut homeostasis possible. Symptoms of candida overgrowth include autoimmune illnesses, persistent digestion problems, chronic nail and skin fungal infections, skin irritation and rashes like eczema and dermatitis, vaginal and/or rectal itching or infection, lack of focus, memory issues, severe seasonal allergies, and cravings for sweets and simple carbs.

ASK THE EXPERTS

For people with SIBO, it is important to wait 3 to 4 hours between meals and avoid snacking. During the digestive process, your small intestine has what are called "cleansing waves," which help push food down to the large intestine between meals. Constant snacking will overload your intestine, and the waves will not be effective in purging your system of excess bacteria.

—Wendie Schneider, RDN

Gut Homeostasis and Liver Function

Happy and balanced microbiota affect the entire body, and your liver is no exception. Your liver is a part of the digestive system and performs a number of critical functions. After the intestine absorbs nutrients during digestion, the liver stores some of them (like vitamin A and iron) and processes others so they can be used throughout the body's other systems. The liver produces chemicals necessary to clot the blood and acts as the blood's filter. It regulates the amount of sugar, protein, and fat in the blood. It breaks down alcohol and other drugs that may enter your system and removes toxins from your blood.

This versatile organ is vital to maintain life, but it's dangerously susceptible to malfunction and disease if the gut is not working symbiotically with its microbiota. Imbalance in the gut can cause a breach in the intestinal lining, introducing pathogens to the bloodstream. The liver filters and sometimes stores the overflow of these pathogens. The by-products of bacterial metabolism play a critical role in the development of liver disease. Similar to a pool with a malfunctioning filter, a malfunctioning liver means the entire body becomes polluted.

Regulating Intake of Common Triggers

So what's the bottom line on achieving and maintaining gut homeostasis? It's all about optimizing the health and diversity of your intestinal microbiota, so they work with your body in perfect symbiosis. One of the best things you can do to ensure this happens is to avoid the eight major culprits (previously listed in the section, "How We Damage Our Tiny Ecosystems") and specifically regulate the intake of common food triggers that cause imbalances in gut bacteria populations.

Here are some common triggers of microbiota imbalance:

Chlorinated drinking water: Chlorine may kill pathogens, but it also kills off healthy gut bacteria.

Simple carbs and sugar: These promote candida and pathogen overgrowth. Many simple carbs also contain gluten, which can throw many gut ecosystems out of whack.

Mass-produced nonorganic animal products: Modern conventional farming practices include the regular use of low-dose antibiotics and low-quality livestock feed.

Genetically modified organisms (GMOs): Genetically engineered foods sometimes contain harmful chemical residue from farming practices; these chemicals destroy gut microbes, especially the beneficial ones.

There is an undeniable link between diet, gut microbiota, and your immune system. Emerging science is just beginning to unravel the intricacies of this relationship between us and the tiny ecosystem we host. They help us absorb vital nutrients and ensure the health of our intestinal wall. One thing is becoming clear: the type of food you eat helps determine the health and optimal functioning of that ecosystem and its role in gut homeostasis.

The Least You Need to Know

- You gut is inhabited by a diverse population of microbes that contribute to digestive and immune function.
- Toxins, stress, poor nutrition, and certain medications can alter the balance of your gut and lead to health problems and a compromised immune system.
- Beneficial bacteria in your gut communicate with your intestinal wall to fight off and contain infection.
- A healthy population of gut microbes can be cultivated by eating a healthy diet and avoiding environmental toxins.

Getting a Diagnosis

You now have some gut basics under your belt and have gained a better understanding of how your digestive system functions. But even experts seek the advice and care of other experts, especially when it comes to matters of health. Putting what you learn into practice often means knowing when it's time to assemble a team of specialists who can diagnose gut-related health conditions and help you develop a plan that integrates nutrition, fitness, lifestyle, and medical interventions where appropriate.

In this chapter, you learn when and how to seek professional counseling for gut issues. We outline the fields of expertise relevant to helping you achieve optimal gut health. We also give you advice about how to work with these individuals as an educated patient.

In This Chapter

- Knowing when gut issues warrant professional intervention
- Assembling your medical team
- The importance of a holistic approach to a healthy gut
- Useful diagnostic tools and tests for gut-related conditions

When to Seek Help

We all experience temporary changes in how digestion feels from time to time. But the key word in that last sentence is *temporary*. You should be experiencing painless, effortless, brown to green, smooth, S-shaped bowel movements one to three times a day. Your urine should be clear or very light yellow. You shouldn't feel so bloated all the time that you can only wear elastic pants. Heartburn shouldn't accompany every meal.

In short, the daily tasks of eating and going to the bathroom shouldn't feel like daunting emergencies, nor should the colors coming out of your body be shocking or mysterious. These are the most obvious of gut-based symptoms. But sometimes people suffer from other symptoms and conditions with root causes that really lie in the gut. Any prolonged discomfort or symptoms for which there isn't any obvious cause should be a red flag that leads to consultation with a healthcare practitioner.

Disruption of Daily Life and Health

You may already know you have an underlying disease or condition that compromises your health and happiness. If you're happy with the way your treatment has gone so far, than continue on your current path. But since you're reading this book, you're probably looking for additional assistance. If you suffer from chronic mental, skin, or autoimmune disorders and your doctor has never discussed the possible connection to your gut, then talk openly to other doctors and nutritional experts about your options.

Once you've acknowledged a gut-based problem is diminishing your ability to get the most out of life, then you've demonstrated you care enough about your health to change. Conducting research on your symptoms and looking for health professionals in your area are good first steps. The next step is to actually talk to those professionals. That often means putting your embarrassment aside and thinking about everything you have to gain. A correct diagnosis and sound medical advice lead to healthy nutrition and lifestyle choices.

The bottom line about seeking professional help—if the joys and comfort of everyday living are disrupted by gut abnormality and its associated health problems, talk to a doctor. No one should simply suffer in silence and feel there is nothing they can do about their digestive health. Incredible advances have been made in diagnosing and treating gut disorders just in the past few years. If you've tried addressing a gut problem in the past to no avail, consider trying again. The science is continually improving. Find doctors and other practitioners who keep abreast of current studies, and you'll have a team of people who can help you get to the core of your issues and on the way to more optimal gut health.

Unhealthy Gut Symptoms

If your gut has been unhealthy for some time, you may have become accustomed to feeling bad. When feeling poorly and enduring unusual and/or painful symptoms is your "normal," it's especially important to review the signs of a malfunctioning digestive system and gut-based conditions so you can properly evaluate yourself. If you have any of the following symptoms, seek a doctor's advice.

- Persistent loss of appetite not due to a short-term intestinal virus

- Nausea, vomiting not due to a short-term intestinal virus

- Ongoing weight loss not due to purposeful dieting and exercise

- Persistent bowel habit changes like chronic diarrhea and constipation or pain with a bowel movement

- Chronic indigestion and/or heartburn

- Abdominal pain, especially if associated with mealtime

- Excessive bloating and flatulence

- Painful or difficult swallowing

- Black, tarry, or bloody stools, or stools containing mucus

- Lack of energy and/or fever accompanied by abdominal symptoms

None of these symptoms is acceptable, and all of them are treatable. Again, adopt the attitude that you will not suffer in silence. Even if the symptom is embarrassing to you, reach out for help. Digestive discomfort does not have to be a part of your daily routine.

As we've discussed, for some people, symptoms of an unhealthy gut manifest in other parts of the body. Food allergies and intolerances, asthma, autoimmune disorders, skin conditions, and even mental illness can all start with gut imbalances and malfunctioning. If you suffer from any of these ailments and have never considered the gut connection before, consider reevaluating your current approach to treating your symptoms.

Success Story

From a patient of Wendie Schneider, RDN

Elizabeth S. suffered from allergies and eczema her whole life. She grew up taking medications, steroids, and creams to try to gain relief from the horrible symptoms. At the age of 34, she came in to my office for weight loss, and had dermatitis around her nose and mouth. Her face burned and was very painful to wash. What she did not realize was that she had nutrient deficiencies, food sensitivities, a damaged gut, and product sensitivities.

She began to use natural face products. She was put on a gut protocol that included taking probiotics to restore and heal the gut. Her body had become so sensitive that whenever she ate sugar, wheat, or sauces her face would flare up. She followed a very strict diet to eliminate the food allergens, and filled her body with the nutrients she was missing. Within 2 weeks, her body experienced a dramatic healing. Just 2 weeks of eating nourishing, whole foods changed her skin more than years of medications and steroid creams.

As time moved on, her digestive system became stronger and she no longer had severe reactions to foods that she had been sensitive to before. She can now, incrementally and in small portions, fit most foods back into her diet. She now understands the importance of managing her body through eating whole foods, getting enough sleep, and managing her stress.

Assembling Your Medical Team

Attaining optimal gut health means being willing to do your homework and reach out to the appropriate medical professionals. Just as with every other endeavor in life, success is never really achieved in isolation. We all need a team that has our best interests at heart. You, however, are in charge of assembling that team.

Too often, people hold medical practitioners on a pedestal and believe they are infallible, and their every recommendation and prescription is gospel—not to be questioned. While it is certainly true that medical professionals are highly educated specialists whose advice certainly holds more water than the layman's, they are also human. You know your own health goals. So to achieve them, you may have to go out of your way to find dedicated and trained individuals who will help you on your journey toward healing your gut and living life to the fullest.

Your Primary Care Physician

When you read advice in this book that prompts you to "seek medical advice" or "see a doctor," what does that mean? What we mean is to consult with your primary care physician. This is not just a random doctor you meet in a one-off visit to an urgent care center. Don't get us wrong. Those facilities have their place, such as when you're on vacation or when your regular doctor's office is closed. But the emergency room or urgent care center is no replacement for the ongoing relationship you should cultivate with a primary care physician (PCP).

GUT WISE

In the age of the internet, there's no reason to fly by the seat of your pants when it comes to choosing a health-care provider. Use websites like Consumer Reports, Yelp, and Zocdoc to help you in your search for a primary care physician that meets your needs and expectations. Don't just read the best and worst reviews and make snap judgments. Read what the majority of patients say about the doctor and make an educated decision.

In the best circumstances, a PCP should be the coordinator of your nonemergency health care. He or she knows your life health history and communicates with any specialists you see. Your PCP is your first point of contact for non-life-threatening medical care and helps to coordinate any more specialized care you might require. This person is usually a medical doctor, but can also be a physician assistant (PA) or nurse practitioner (NP). PAs and NPs are licensed and also require medical school and extensive hands-on training, just not as much as a medical doctor (MD).

A good PCP tends to your long-term health, preventive care, and lifestyle counseling, so it's important to choose one carefully. You want to make sure they accept your insurance, so they're an affordable option for you. You also want to be sure they have a friendly staff and are easy to reach by phone and email. Check their office hours to make sure they're compatible with your schedule.

Meet with a provider before you sign on as a new patient. People often forget this option. You can actually interview the doctor first to be sure you get a good feeling about them. That initial meeting is also a good time to ask about his/her experience with nutrition and gut health.

All this may seem like nitpicking, but ideally your relationship with a PCP is one for the "long haul." You'll be less likely to call and make necessary appointments if your experiences at the doctor's office are inconvenient, annoying, or generally unpleasant. Your main goal is to find a PCP who is on board with preventive help, who has an excellent bedside manner, is easy to talk to, and one who is well versed in nutrition as a means to achieving gut health and addressing other gut-based illnesses.

Choosing a Gastroenterologist

If you have chronic GI issues, your PCP might refer you to a *gastroenterologist* for more intensive and specialized treatment and care. Gastroenterology is the branch of medicine that deals specifically with the stomach and the intestines. There are some issues a PCP may feel are beyond their area of expertise. If the scope of your problem needs intensive management and intervention, you may find yourself in the office of a gastroenterologist.

Our goal is to help you cultivate the healthiest gut possible, and to that end, let us offer general advice on choosing a gastroenterologist. You want to find someone who is open to nutrition as a viable option in treating the underlying causes of stomach and intestinal conditions. Don't get us wrong, medication is often needed, and certain medical procedures are life-saving (especially preventive diagnostic tests like *endoscopies* and *colonoscopies* that can detect ulcers and cancers.) But if you're in a doctor's office and the practitioner simply shrugs off the possibility that diet affects gut health, or doesn't have time to talk with you about probiotics and healing your gut, then it might be time to choose another doctor.

> **DEFINITION**
>
> A **gastroenterologist** is a medical specialist in the digestive system. A **colonoscopy** is a medical diagnostic procedure, usually performed by a gastroenterologist, which detects abnormalities in the rectum and large intestine (colon). It involves the insertion of a tiny camera fixed to the end of a long tube into the anus and colon. In this way, the medical staff can evaluate the health of the last section of your GI tract. The National Cancer Institute recommends everyone undergo a diagnostic colonoscopy at age 50. **Endoscopies** use similar tools as colonoscopies to examine your upper-digestive tract from your throat to the small intestine.

This is not to say that you are looking for doctors who always agree with you and only go along with your point of view. But you are now an empowered patient looking for a team of open-minded medical practitioners who believe in treating the whole patient. You deserve a doctor who has the time to listen to your concerns and counsel you on nutrition as well as write a prescription should it prove necessary. You deserve a gastroenterologist well versed in the emerging science of the brain-gut axis, the roll of microbiota in overall health, and in the best ways to achieve optimal gut health.

Given the nature of gastroenterology, people are often embarrassed about even seeking an appointment with one. Rest assured these doctors usually choose this specialty because either they or their family members have GI issues, and they were inspired to do something about GI health in general. Still, talking about stomach and bowel troubles is an uncomfortable conversation for some people. Here are some tips to keep in mind once you choose a GI specialist, so you can talk to your doctor without dying from embarrassment:

Perspective: Is it worth risking your health for a few moments of potential blushing? They've heard it before. Really. They have.

Full disclosure: Your doctor is a professional doctor, not a mind reader. You have to tell him/her about your symptoms.

Be proactive: Go for an annual healthy check-up so you're not nervous when you go just when something is wrong.

Be comfortable in your own skin: No one likes stripping down to a paper gown, but you may have to if you're going for bowel troubles. Be prepared so you don't chicken out about discussing a crucial symptom you have. Shower, shave, and wear your best socks and underwear. In short, don't give yourself excuses for why you didn't get properly examined.

Use your own words: Don't worry about technical jargon—that's the doctor's job. If you can't remember the medical term for anatomy or bodily function, just say the words you know. Every gastroenterologist has said and heard the word *poop*.

Write it down: If you feel like saying any of this out loud would be too mortifying, then write it all down before you go and hand the doctor a note. I guarantee you wouldn't be the first.

Nutritionists and Dietitians

Some people use the terms *nutritionist* and *dietitian* interchangeably. While both types of practitioners can offer similar counseling, there are important distinctions between the two in terms of qualifications, licensing, regulation, and expertise levels. It's important to keep these differences in mind when assembling the best health team possible.

A dietitian is someone who has completed a BS in nutrition or *dietetics* or obtained an MS in those subjects after first completing an undergraduate degree in science. Part of a dietitian's training is practical medical field training, so they are fully qualified to advise patients in therapeutic nutrition. The title of "dietitian" is granted only after the completion of accredited degree programs and their accompanying practical training. Additionally, dietitians take certified board examinations. A registered dietitian must complete continuing education credits to maintain a license and registration each year.

DEFINITION

Dietitians are experts in nutrition with degrees in science, practical training, and board certification. **Dietetics** is the study of nutrition and its effect on the body.

Dietitians are qualified to work in hospital or community settings to provide scientifically sound advice about food. They offer nutrition advice to those with medical conditions and help diagnose food-related illnesses and those illness that can be treated with diet, including diseases that begin in the gut. The term *registered dietitian* means the practitioner is a member of a professional organization and is accountable for his or her actions as a health-care provider.

A nutritionist is someone who has completed coursework in nutrition. But because the title isn't accredited, virtually anyone can call themselves a nutritionist. Some nutritionists have substantial training and qualifications and work in the food and health sectors. They may have degrees in food science or nutrition. As nutritionists, however, they are not required to undergo accredited practical training in a medical environment and are not qualified to diagnose or treat diseases.

ASK THE EXPERTS

Your RDN dietitian can help you determine which foods are triggering your symptoms, how to build a balanced diet without those foods (or in limited quantities), and what to look for on food labels or when dining out. For many, completely omitting a food or food group is unnecessary and can be unhealthy. Striking a balance between eating enough for the nutritional benefits and not too much to trigger symptoms can be tricky. This is where a knowledgeable dietitian comes in. Make sure your dietitian has the RD or RDN credential behind his or her name.

—Kristen Tice-Ziesmer, MS, RD, CSSD, LD, sports dietitian, ACE-certified personal trainer, owner of Elite Nutrition and Performance

Most dietitians identify themselves as "registered dietitian nutritionists" to affirm they are qualified experts in the field of nutrition. In this way, all dietitians are nutritionists, but not all nutritionists are dietitians. For the purposes of a healthy gut, a dietitian (an RD or RDN) is your best bet. These professionals will help you evaluate your food habits, diagnose, and manage any food-related intolerances or allergies you might have, and diagnose and manage gut-related conditions. They are well versed in using nutrition to achieve optimal gut health.

Integrative Medicine

One of the most exciting and promising trends in health care is the rise of *integrative medicine.* This field adopts a patient-centered approach. Attentive and mindful doctors have always taken this path, but now more than ever there is a growing consensus that the best way to address a patient's health is by taking into consideration the entire spectrum of factors that influence our health. These factors include physical, mental, emotional, environmental, and even spiritual elements.

GUT WISE

Finding a good doctor in your area can be a daunting task, especially if you want to limit the use of pharmaceuticals and treat the root cause of the symptoms. This type of doctor is called an Integrative Physician. If you are looking for this type of doctor try these websites: functionalmedicine.org, naturopathic.org, or acamnet.org. Make sure you find a doctor who works with other doctors and is a team player; can discuss lifestyle changes such as sleep, nutrition, and stress; and can answer "why" if you have questions about any prescribed tests or drugs.

Another term included in this idea is *complementary and alternative medicine* (CAM), which the National Institutes of Health (NIH) define as healing modalities, therapies, philosophies, or approaches that are outside of mainstream use in Western medicine. Notice the term *complementary,* which means "in addition to" or "combining in a way that enhances another existing element." Complementary and alternative medicine, when used in conjunction with conventional Western medical knowledge, provides a broad spectrum of approaches that can address all the underlying factors that influence gut health.

The National Center for Complementary and Alternative Medicine (NCCAM) divide CAM into five categories:

Mind-body medicine: Examines and treats the way our brain and emotional states influence physical health. An example of this in practice would be treating the way emotional trauma can cause GI problems by engaging in meditation as a means of stress management.

Whole medical systems: Include older non-Western schools of medical practice such an ancient Chinese and Indian traditions.

Manipulative and body-based practices: Include physical movement of the body to improve health, such as chiropractic treatment.

Energy medicine: Uses the energy fields that some practitioners believe encircle the body. Examples of energy medicine include acupuncture and magnet therapy.

Biologically based practices: Focus on nutrition and herbal remedies.

Whether or not you're open to a more integrative approach to health care is a matter of personal preference and comfort level. Having more options in addressing your gut health concerns can seem daunting. But if you've tried basic conventional medicine and your doctor doesn't ask you prying questions about basic influences like what you're eating, daily stress levels, and exercise habits, then consider a more holistic approach.

> **DEFINITION**
>
> **Integrative medicine** is a patient-centered approach to health care that takes into account physical, psychological, social, environmental, and spiritual influences at work in their lives. **Complementary and alternative medicine** includes both conventional and nonconventional (and traditionally non-Western) approaches to health care.

There are many open-minded PCPs who are part of health-care groups that offer talk therapy, dietary counseling, and acupuncture or who would at least refer you to a trusted CAM practitioner. Knowing what we know about the brain-gut axis, and that knowledge continues to deepen, it really isn't far-fetched to think CAM methods could be helpful in overcoming some of the more debilitating or persistent symptoms of an unhealthy gut.

Personal Trainers

The link between exercise and overall well-being is clear and proven. But consider the specific effects of exercise and GI health. Regular moderate exercise improves circulation and brain function, and we already know how important these connections are to the bodily functions involved in digestion. A regularly moving body means a regularly moving GI tract, which helps promote healthy digestion and bowel movements.

You know that exercise is good for you, but maybe you're not motivated enough to do it. A personal trainer can give you specialized advice, attention, and the accountability you need to stick with an exercise regimen. If you know you'll need someone to "kick your butt" to get you to exercise, then a personal trainer might be a good option for you.

You don't have to be mega-rich to enjoy the services of a good personal trainer. Gyms often employ their own staff to work with members at reasonable fees, at least in the introductory phase. If you know you can stick to a program once you've learned it, then consider signing up for just a few sessions. Sometimes all you need is someone to get you started, suggest certain workouts, and show you the correct form for the best exercises to accomplish your fitness goals.

As a side note: in 2014, scientists discovered that rigorous exercise may play a role in promoting diverse gut bacteria populations. Therefore, the more diverse your population, the more chances you have for a robust and flourishing inner ecosystem that boosts your immunity and your brain-axis communications.

The caveat we offer for finding a nutritionist also applies to finding a personal trainer. As with the title "nutritionist," anyone can call himself a "personal trainer." You need to seek out someone with a fitness certification from a program accredited by an independent, third-party organization. One well-respected third-party accreditation service is the National Commission for Certifying Agencies (NCCA).

> **GUT WISE**
>
> Many personal trainers offer specific nutrition advice to their clients, but they shouldn't. Personal trainers can state facts, but they shouldn't prescribe nutritional specifics. Anything beyond general recommendations should be given by someone with more education such as a registered dietitian. Acceptable: "Chicken is a good source of protein." Not acceptable: "You should be eating 16 ounces of chicken per day." There is a distinct difference between sharing general information and making prescriptive suggestions. Talk to a dietitian or nutritionist before making any changes to your diet.

Testing

After you've assembled your team of qualified health-care professionals, the real work of diagnosis can begin. Sometimes an anecdotal recounting of your symptoms will be enough, so be sure to be forthcoming about your symptoms and honestly answer all of the practitioner's questions. If mere physical exam and symptom-checking aren't enough, however, there are several tests available to pinpoint the cause of gut problems.

Most of the testing involves an in-depth analysis of your blood. Clinicians can evaluate whether or not you have nutrient deficiencies and prescribe ways you can correct those deficits. Food sensitivities can also be determined by bloodwork. Gut bacteria imbalance can be detected by a range of breath tests, urinalysis, and stool samples. There are options out there, and your professional team can help you get to the root of your gut ailments.

Basic Physical

Gut health is often a barometer of how the rest of the body is functioning. One of the best tools you have at your disposal in maintaining your health, and diagnosing and treating underlying conditions, is to establish a good relationship with a PCP and receive a basic physical about every year, even when you're feeling great. This will establish your baselines and norms so your doctor can note any marked changes.

Recently some discrepancies have emerged in the general medical community about how often patients should undergo basic physical exams. The frequency of these "healthy visits" will depend on your age, previous health history, and the recommendations of your PCP and other specialists you may see, like a gastroenterologist. Once a year is a good idea for achieving and maintaining optimal gut health.

A basic physical exam consists of updating your health history, which will include a list of medications and supplements as well as lifestyle factors like a new job and the status of the major relationships in your life. Your blood pressure, heart and respiratory rate are checked, which will give you one indication of how your diet impacts other body systems. The doctor should also give you a visual once-over and check the condition of your skin, nails, hair, limbs, and abdominal area for any changes that might indicate a problem—another indicator of the state of your diet's impact on the body.

Physical exams should also be accompanied by a complete blood count and chemistry panel (CBC). These tests show abnormalities in the blood indicative of health conditions, cholesterol levels, and other factors your doctor deems important. Family history will indicate the age at which a doctor may want to screen you for certain cancers, bone diseases, and diabetes.

Detecting Vitamin and Mineral Deficiencies

In Chapter 2, we discussed some symptoms of vitamin and mineral deficiencies and how a malfunctioning small and large intestine can lead to poor nutrient absorption. If symptoms of suspected vitamin or mineral deficiencies are persistent problems, your doctor or dietitian could perform a blood test to determine the exact deficiency and prescribe an appropriate nutrition regimen or supplement to correct it.

To review, persistent fatigue, loss of appetite, unexplained and unintentional weight loss, muscle cramps, pain, weakness, abnormal heartbeat, increase in minor and severe infections, bone pain, vomiting, diarrhea, constipation, excessive unwarranted sweating, coordination and balance issues, anemia, brain fog, and numbness in the extremities may be signs of vitamin or mineral deficiencies and can be pinpointed by blood tests. There are many micronutrient blood panels available for you and your doctor to request. Keep in mind, however, that insurance might not cover all of them. It will depend on the severity of your symptoms and your doctor's rationale for ordering the tests. The bureaucracy of the insurance system is a confounding beast, but keep in mind that your gut health is crucial.

If you're simply curious about whether or not your body is absorbing certain nutrients, chances are you're footing the bill on your own. But that doesn't mean the results aren't useful to you. You'll know for sure if your diet and nutritional regimen are providing you with everything your gut needs. You may want to go the extra mile and request "cellular analysis" in addition to a regular blood test. Cellular analysis provides details about the presence, absorption, and effectiveness of the micronutrients in your body. In a regular blood test, the mere presence of the nutrient can't measure whether or not the nutrient is benefitting your cells and contributing to functions like immunity.

The IgG, IgE, IgM, and IgA Panels

Your body's immune system produces proteins to fight off antigens—threats introduced to the body like pathogenic bacteria, viruses, and toxins. These proteins are called antibodies or *immunoglobulins*. Once your body comes into contact with an antigen and produces an antibody to fight it, that pattern becomes a learned and repeated response. Your immune system will keep making those antibodies. This is how our body fights off disease.

> **DEFINITION**
>
> Your immune system makes specialized proteins called **immunoglobulins** to fight off invaders in the body. These proteins are also called antibodies.

A blood test that measures the immunoglobulins in your blood can help a doctor determine if your immune system is functioning properly. It can also reveal if you have infections or immune system dysfunction due to malnutrition, autoimmune conditions (such as rheumatoid arthritis, lupus, or celiac disease), or food allergies to common triggers like gluten and dairy. There are four types of antibodies doctors will commonly test for:

Immunoglobulin A (IgA): An antibody found in the lining of the GI tract, nasal cavities, and lungs.

Immunoglobulin G (IgG): The antibody found in every body fluid; it protects against infections.

Immunoglobulin M (IgM): Your body's "first-responder" to infections; it's like a microscopic paramedic that lives in your blood and lymphatic fluid.

Immunoglobulin E (IgE): Found in the membranes of skin, lungs, and mucosal cells and is associated with allergic reactions.

The results of these types of blood tests can help you determine if your immune system is out of whack and if you have a previously undiagnosed autoimmune disorder. Your doctor may also order addition panels to determine your overall immune function, such as Th1 and Th2 cytokine blood panels that deal with white blood cell analysis. Blood test results can help you make adjustments in your diet to boost your immune system, rectify underlying conditions, and balance your gut bacteria population to be on your way to a healthier gut.

SIBO Testing

Small intestinal bacterial overgrowth (SIBO) can happen when nerve or muscle damage in the intestines prevents the normal movement of bacteria from the small to the large intestine that occurs with normal digestion. If too many bacteria are left in the small intestines after the food passes through, the bacteria population explodes and the gut microbiota are out of balance. Preexisting medical conditions and their accompanying medications can also cause SIBO. Antacids, antibiotics, steroids, and alcohol can all disrupt the gut flora.

If you have food intolerances, excess gas, IBS, or undiagnosed abdominal discomfort, a dietitian, PCP, or gastroenterologist can test you for SIBO. Sometimes a practitioner will treat you for SIBO simply by knowing your medical history and listening to your symptoms. Other times, exact tests are needed. There are three major tests to determine if SIBO is present:

Breath test: Requires you to fast for 12 hours ahead of time. In the doctor's office you then breathe into a balloon, eat a measured amount of sugar, and continue to give breath samples into the balloon every 15 minutes for around 3 hours.

Organix Dysbiosis test: Is a urine test that measures the by-products of bacteria and yeast.

Comprehensive stool test (fecal culture): Requires a stool sample that will measure the levels of bacteria in the large intestine.

If you have SIBO, it's often treated with the antibiotic Xifaxan. But knowing what you know about antibiotics, you may want to try to balance your gut flora by changing your diet first. Talk to your doctor openly about your concerns. Often a diet that is free from simple carbs, sugars, alcohol, and gluten can help resolve SIBO over time. These are some of the same principles we discuss in Part 3.

Extreme Cases: Fecal Transplants

Fecal cultures (stool sample analysis) shed light on the composition of your gut bacteria population. If your gut is overpopulated by the pathogenic strain *Clostridium difficile,* then your health is in serious decline. This nasty strain of bacteria causes chronic diarrhea. In 2012, 14,000 people died of from C. difficile in the United States alone. The most successful treatment for this overgrowth is a fecal microbiota transplant or FMT. There is also a promising future for the use of FMT in the treatment of autoimmune conditions, including IBS, Crohn's, and ulcerative colitis.

FMTs are performed by mixing feces from a healthy donor with balanced gut flora, mixing the feces with a saline solution, and then placing the mixture into the sick patient with a tube inserted into the anus, much like a colonoscopy procedure. The gross-out factor may relegate this treatment to the realm of "all things taboo" for a lot of people, but there's actually a lot of history behind its use. The first documented fecal transplant was in fourth-century China. Since then, there have been no serious side effects reported with the procedure. It will be interesting to see how it's used to help more people overcome gut issues by completely repopulating their gut microbiota.

The Least You Need to Know

- If persistent GI symptoms or undiagnosed health conditions prevent you from enjoying life, it's time to seek medical help.
- Assemble a team of health practitioners and make informed decisions about treatment, nutrition, and other lifestyle choices under their care.
- A solid relationship with an open-minded primary care physician is crucial to gut health and general well-being.
- Educate yourself about diagnostic tests that determine underlying conditions, food sensitivities, allergies, and gut imbalance.

Understanding Leaky Gut Syndrome

More than 2,000 years ago, Hippocrates famously stated, "all disease begins in the gut." Emerging science is proving that's a pretty accurate statement. The connections between your gut and your overall health are undeniable.

In this part, we unpack the mystery of intestinal hyperpermeability, also known as "leaky gut syndrome." We examine how what you eat can impact your body right down to your DNA. Food and lifestyle choices have a dramatic impact on your gastrointestinal health, which in turn affects the rest of your body. A leaky gut can become a vicious cycle aggravated by the use of common medications and the consumption of food that further damage the lining of your intestines. We examine the common pitfalls in the typical diet and modern living that take a toll on your gut.

Part 2 shows you how you can apply current scientific knowledge about leaky gut to help you make better choices and keep your gut healthy.

CHAPTER 5

Gut Hyperpermeability and the Medical Consensus

We often use phrases to discuss bad food choices like, "that didn't agree with me" or "that upset my stomach" as if our GI tract had a mind and personality of its own. Well, in a way it does. We've already discussed the brain-gut axis and the role the enteric nervous system and your gut bacteria play in your immunity. Your gut, and specifically your small intestine, plays an enormous role in your overall health. If your small intestine isn't happy, that unease is going to play out elsewhere in your body. How does small intestine damage spread to other places in the body? Leaky gut syndrome.

In this chapter, we define leaky gut syndrome and its underlying causes. You learn the science that led to understanding intestinal permeability and what we now know about the way autoimmune diseases develop in the body as a result of a damaged intestinal lining. We delve into the medical community's response to leaky gut. We'll also examine how new advances in genetics show us how we can take control of our health, even if we have the genetic markers for diseases that begin in the gut.

In This Chapter

- The causes and effects of intestinal hyperpermeability
- Why some dismiss leaky gut
- How your diet turns genes on and off in your body
- Ways integrative medicine helps address intestinal hyperpermeability

What Is Leaky Gut Syndrome?

The term *leaky gut* is often used to describe intestinal permeability, or more specifically, *hyper-permeability*. During the past 30 years, scientists have discovered that the cells in the intestinal wall are held together by tight junctions—specialized connectors that operate like swinging doors. Most of the time they're shut, but the body and its invaders have mechanisms, like secret passwords, that cause them to swing open. Tight junctions allow small particles to be released into the circulatory system. This is a good pathway if the particle is a health-inducing molecule the body needs, a bad pathway if it's an undigested bit of food or strain of harmful bacteria.

Tight junctions communicate with certain proteins, as well as your gut bacteria, in order to keep the intestinal lining intact and to perform its two main jobs: absorbing nutrients and keeping pathogens in check. When we eat foods that "upset the stomach," the lining can become overly porous, and our first line of immune defense in the gut sets off chain reactions elsewhere in the body. This series of events often leads to disease, or at the very least, worsens existing symptoms that we might already have.

But if we feed our body right, we can keep the bad *genes* from activating by keeping antigens (the "bad stuff") from entering the bloodstream in the first place. Eating well also keeps gut bacteria populations in balance and enhances the effectiveness of the immune system whose headquarters lie smack dab in the middle of our gut. Preventing excessive intestinal permeability starts with an understanding of what causes it, what aggravates it, and what can reverse it.

The Role of Zonulin and Gut Permeability

Until the 1980s, we didn't know about tight junctions. And when scientists discovered them, they still didn't understand what mechanisms caused them to open and close. Then, in April 2000, Dr. Alessio Fasano and his team of researchers at the University of Maryland announced they'd discovered a protein in the human body whose job was to regulate the opening of tight junctions between the cells that line the small intestine. They called this protein *zonulin*, and it was the missing piece of the tight-junction-function puzzle.

 DEFINITION

> **Genes** are made up of strands of DNA molecules that instruct individual body cells to make different proteins they need to form and function. Your genes are inherited and passed on to the next generation. **Zonulin** is a protein that controls the opening and closing of tight junctions in the gut lining.

Zonulin actually causes tight junctions to open. This process helps with the active transport of nutrients into the circulatory system. But, as with everything else in life, having too much of a good thing causes problems. There are two factors that cause the cells that line our intestines to release excess amounts of zonulin: small intestinal bacterial overgrowth (SIBO) and exposure to *gliadin,* a protein found in gluten.

No matter who you are, SIBO and gluten will open your tight junctions and release material into your bloodstream. Whether this reaction is harmful depends on your genetics. If you have a healthy immune system and no genes for autoimmune illness, your body will flush out the bad bacteria and handle the gluten without you even being aware of it. But if you're prewired to have a more hypersensitive immune system, your body is going to overreact to undigested gluten and bacteria and cause inflammation.

GUT WISE

Elevated levels of zonulin are associated with celiac disease, Crohn's disease, irritable bowel disease (IBD), Type 1 diabetes, multiple sclerosis, asthma, and other inflammatory and autoimmune disorders. It is especially important that people with these disorders ensure they take some form of probiotics. The quality and ratio of good to bad gut bacteria are important, even more so in people with high zonulin levels that will suffer from hyperpermeable intestinal walls. Probiotic supplements and those in fermented foods are a good first step toward healing the gut.

Dr. Fasano's Research

Like many other major scientific breakthroughs, the discovery of zonulin came when it wasn't expected. Dr. Fasano was actually working on a vaccine for cholera when he discovered how zonulin works to regulate the opening and closing of tight junctions between the enterocytes of the intestinal wall. What he discovered was a game changer for treating celiac disease and laid the groundwork for treating other autoimmune diseases as well.

Fasano's team revealed that people with celiac and other autoimmune diseases produce excess zonulin. But we don't want to demonize the protein. After all, it regulates the passage of white blood cells and proteins in and out of the intestine. It's also an important communicator between the gut and our immune system. Zonulin is like the automatic garage door opener that lets you safely park your car in a protected space. However, you wouldn't want the automatic opener to trigger your garage door to open at 3 A.M. when a known felon was on the loose in your neighborhood.

Zonulin is only problematic if its levels get too high. When that happens, it's as if the garage door will open for anybody at any time. Then the body is being flooded by gluten or other antigens on a regular basis. If a person has the genes for autoimmune responses, those genes will gear up and program the immune system to respond. A microbiota imbalance will only exacerbate the response. When all of those factors come together, a negative cycle perpetuates itself like a bad cold that runs through a classroom all season long—there's constant exposure, so there's constant "reinfection."

This negative cycle explains how autoimmune diseases have their root in leaky gut syndrome. The damaged intestinal lining continually allows foreign substances into the body. The liver, the body's main filter, can't handle the overload of toxins. The immune system struggles to launch attack after attack but can't keep up. A battle-fatigued body is more prone to infection. A stressed immune system can't fight off every single antigen, so some of them absorb into body tissue. Constant antigen presence signals even more immune attacks and *autoimmunity* is born— damaging healthy tissue with widespread inflammation.

> **DEFINITION**
>
> Gluten contains a protein called **gliadin,** which triggers the production and often overproduction of zonulin in the intestine. The combination of immune responses that result in an organism's immune system attacking its own healthy tissues is called **autoimmunity.**

Acceptance in the Medical Community

Dr. Fasano's team proved the theory of excessive intestinal permeability. Their work on celiac disease demonstrated something that had previously confused the medical community. Doctors knew their celiac patients developed autoimmunity to gluten. But how did that gluten get directly into the system? That's not how the body is supposed to operate. Individual proteins and nutrients are delivered through the intestinal wall via passive and active transport. Undigested food particles aren't supposed to get through. Yet eliminating gluten from a celiac's diet relieved nearly all a patient's symptoms. Why?

Fasano's team provided the answer. Overproduction of zonulin leaves the tight junctions *wide* open for prolonged periods, allowing antigens (in the case of celiac disease, gluten) to be directly introduced to the immune system. Once in the bloodstream, antigen presence also provides the opportunity for genetic predisposition to kick into gear. The body of the celiac, whose DNA is already prewired to be sensitive to gluten, mounts an antibody attack against the healthy tissue of the gut.

GUT WISE

In 2000, the *New England Journal of Medicine* released a paper about the negative effects of blue dye when added tube feeding formulas in the ICU. This was a common practice for feeding patients through their gut in hospitals until this time. The dye would show up in patients' tracheal secretions if they accidentally inhaled the contents of their feeding tubes. Deaths were reported because of absorption of the blue dye from the gut to other organs including the skin, blood serum, and urine due to intestinal hyperpermeability.

Between 2000 and 2003, Fasano's team paved the way for other researchers in the field of autoimmunity. There are now hundreds of papers and studies in the medical literature about intestinal permeability and its impact on how the body develops disease. Despite this, there are still some conventional medical doctors who disregard the mounting evidence. Why are they so stubborn?

In their defense, the concept of leaky gut predates Dr. Fasano's research. The idea proliferated among alternative and complementary and alternative medical (CAM) practitioners whom conventional doctors didn't take seriously. The diagnosis of leaky gut was arguably thrown around too loosely, and in this way it lost its credibility with some doctors. With the advent of such discoveries as the role of tight junctions and zonulin, we hope more conventional doctors will accept the fact of intestinal hyperpermeability.

Success Story

S. Jane Gari

In 2007, I was diagnosed with rheumatoid and psoriatic arthritis. The diagnoses didn't come as a shock. I'd known for years that something was wrong with my joints. Like many people, mystery symptoms that were annoying and didn't seem life-threatening got relegated to the back burner.

But after the birth of my daughter, the symptoms became unbearable. My knee joints would become so swollen and painful that I could barely walk at times. Every morning began with running my hands under hot water until I could loosen them enough to make a fist, so I could brush my teeth and wash my face. Even these small tasks would be painful. Most days I couldn't wear my wedding ring.

Something had to give.

continues

continued

I made an appointment with a rheumatologist who prescribed me an indefinite course of steroids in conjunction with other anti-rheumatic and anti-inflammatory drugs. This worked well for controlling flare-ups for about a year. While visiting family out of town, I started to experience intermittent nausea and tarry stools. I chalked it up to being travel-weary until, after 3 days of stomach upset, my heart started racing wildly. Then I lost consciousness. I landed in the ICU for a week due to four bleeding ulcers my prescriptions had caused. After vomiting up 40 percent of my body's blood, I received a life-saving transfusion and resolved to wean myself off the medications.

After I recovered, I sought the counsel of a registered dietician who determined the underlying cause of my RA was intestinal hyperpermeability ("leaky gut") and SIBO. After identifying the triggers that caused my gut and joint inflammation, I no longer needed my medications to live symptom-free. I just needed to heal my gut through diet and probiotic supplementation. When I returned to my rheumatologist to show him my progress, he dismissed the fact that nutrition had helped me achieve near-remission and called it a coincidence. He also gave no credence to intestinal hyper-permeability and balked at the idea of suggesting his patients seek the counsel of dietitians.

My rheumatologist was a kind-hearted man who wanted to help people. But sadly, most conventional doctors receive very little formal training in nutrition while in medi-cal school. Currently, I see my dietitian and my primary care physician to manage my arthritis. These days, managing the disease just means steering clear of the foods that trigger my symptoms and keeping stress in check. (More on how to do that for yourself in Part 3.) My primary care physician goes out of his way to educate himself and his patients about nutrition and lifestyle choices and how they impact the prevention and even treatment of disease. My story truly is one of the successes of integrative medicine.

The Role of Epigenetics

When you hear that you have the gene for a certain disease, it doesn't mean you currently suf-fer active symptoms. The disease is often lying dormant waiting for something to trigger the gene to begin its dark work. *Epigenetics* investigates the mystery of those triggers. Epigenetics is an emerging field of science that studies how the expression of genes in organisms can be changed. In other words, it's the study of what factors can switch genes on or off and how this impacts not only us, but our children and grandchildren. After all, genes are inherited and passed along to the next generation.

Genes are made up of chromosomes. Chromosomes are made up of DNA, which are long, ladder-shaped molecules containing four basic compounds (comprised of bases, sugars, and acids). The different configurations of these four compounds are like programming codes for your body. DNA is the tiny instruction manual inside nearly every cell of your body. All of your body systems take their orders from this genetic material.

So what does epigenetics have to do with gut health specifically? Everything. If your gut lining is damaged and has become hyperpermeable, foreign substances in your system are being introduced to your body's systems. These interactions are opportunities for genes to change the way they express themselves. Simply put, the food you eat, the lifestyle choices you make, and the environmental factors you're exposed to can influence your DNA.

Epigenetics: The Study of Changes in Gene Expression

Traditional genetics used to dictate that if you have a gene for something you are stuck with it—your genes are your destiny. Then the belief evolved into the idea that a gene is like a seed with potential, mysteriously reaching fruition or lying dormant for life. Epigenetics is a more sophisticated study of genes and how they operate. This new science concludes that many genes are highly influenced by environmental factors, such as your dietary and lifestyle choices and exposure to toxins (like heavy metal and molds.) Even stress, surgery, and trauma (like car accidents) can play a role in activating a gene.

Epigenetics dates back to the 1940s. Back then, the science was focused on how genes play a role in our early development. In the 1990s, epigenetic scientists began to investigate how and why genes express themselves, not just during a human's developing years, but throughout our lives. The science now examines which environmental factors cause genes to become active or dormant, specifically when it comes to mental and immune disorders.

Epigenetics also examines the relationship between our microbiota and gene expression. Those bacteria of ours play an important role in almost every bodily function. The rise of more allergies and intestinal problems is in direct correlation with nutrition and lifestyle choices affecting the health of the microbiome in our gut. Major disturbances in the health of our gut bacteria community that lead to intestinal hyperpermeability can compromise the genes in charge of complicated immune system processes.

When the microbiota are out of whack, it affects the *metabolites* that send signals to the brain via the vagus nerve and other pathways. The microbiota also communicate and interact with the epithelial cells of the intestinal wall and cause tight-junction deformity, which leaves large holes in the intestinal barrier. When antigens are released through these holes, they interact with other body systems and our DNA, causing bad genes to go into action.

> **DEFINITION**
>
> **Epigenetics** is the study of how genes express themselves and what factors influence those expressions. **Metabolites** are small molecules produced during metabolism, which includes all the processes necessary for cell generation, growth, survival, and reproduction. The process that regulates gene expression and cell repair is called **methylation.** This occurs when a set of one carbon linked to three hydrogen molecules is given to a molecule.

If you already have a genetic marker that makes your system predisposed to act in a certain way (like an inherited gene for an autoimmune illness), then you're even more vulnerable to these genes expressing negatively when your microbiome is imbalanced. Studies show how leaky gut often flips the genetic on-switch for diseases such as celiac disease, Type 1 diabetes, rheumatoid arthritis, and multiple sclerosis.

Methylation: The Genetic Switch Flipper

So how do these genetic changes actually occur in the body? How does a gene get activated by factors like what we eat? The answer lies in a process called *methylation.* Methylation is the chemistry term for when a molecule gives another molecule a set of atoms: one carbon linked to three hydrogens. Why should we care about this chemistry in the body? When those atoms are exchanged, healing happens. Methylation is a cellular repair process in the body happening at the rate of roughly a billion times a second. It's enormously important.

> **GUT WISE**
>
> Poor methylation can affect bile production. Bile breaks down fats. If we don't have enough bile, our gut bacteria feed on those fats. This could lead to chronic and persistent leaky gut that is difficult to heal without addressing the source of the poor methylation. If you have poor bile production that doesn't resolve with conventional treatment, consider working with a dietitian or another CAM practitioner who can help identify which genes are being expressed. CAM professionals can help treat the issue with specific supplements, nutritional regimens, and even pharmaceutical treatments.

Methylation helps the body detox, controls inflammation, fights viruses, and boosts immunity by aiding in the production of T-cells (those white blood cells that identify foreign invaders and rally the rest of your immune cells to the rescue). Methylation is the process by which genes express themselves.

Methylation also aids in adenosine triphosphate (ATP) production. ATP is the molecule that cells produce to store the energy a cell needs to perform all its functions properly. It's often referred to by biologists as the "energetic currency" of life itself. If methylation helps produce the vital molecule that stores energy every single cell in our body needs to do its job, we should make sure we make choices that ensures that process runs smoothly.

When our gut health is poor, the nutrients getting sent to cells are poor. Without proper nutrition, methylation is mediocre at best. Eating healthy foods is one way we can help methylation influence our genes in the best way possible.

 YOU ARE WHAT YOU EAT

Eating liver and green leafy vegetables helps boost positive methylation.

The Flexibility of Microbiota Genomes

The human body contains approximately 20,000 different genes, all of which play a role in our physical characteristics and the function of cells and organ systems. But good old bacteria's genes outnumber our own by about 100 to 1. Epigenetics is also studying the genes of the bacteria, specifically the bacteria that live in our gut. This population is crucial to maintaining a healthy gut, and science is only just beginning to sequence the genes of the human microbiome.

There is so much we don't yet understand about the exact mechanisms gut bacteria use to communicate with our bodies' systems. We do know, however, that the genes of many beneficial bacteria are highly flexible; they can regularly transfer genetic material among themselves. Whereas humans rely on longer periods in between generations for genetic changes to occur, bacteria don't need to wait. They quickly adapt and change based on their environment. And what we eat has a profound effect on their environment—our GI tract.

Gut bacteria play a role in the early development of the gastrointestinal tract and the growth of a child overall. There are even some foods, like complex plant matter, humans wouldn't be able to digest without the special enzymes certain gut bacteria make. Gut microbes play a significant role throughout our lives in providing us with energy from our food. In this way, gut bacteria communicate with our cells and influence methylation and the way our very genes express themselves.

Epigeneticists and microbiologists are hard at work mapping the genes of the microbiota that live in the human intestines. Understanding exactly how they communicate and influence our bodies, especially the integrity of the intestinal wall, will enhance the effectiveness of probiotics.

Currently, the probiotic supplements you can buy to enhance your gut health are limited. Scientists have only completely mapped out the genes of a few probiotic strains. With around 1,000 species of bacteria living inside your GI tract, it will take many years for medical research to unravel the genetic codes of the human microbiome.

GUT WISE

Scientists have completely mapped the genes for these probiotic gut bacteria: *Bifidobacterium longum, Lactobacillus plantarum, Lactobacillus johnsonii,* and *Lactobacillus acidophilus.*

For now, we have to satisfy ourselves with knowing that the tiny ecosystem inside us is vital to our well-being. We can use the genetic information available on bacteria in choosing a probiotic product if we're diagnosed with SIBO or gut bacteria imbalance. Our microbiota build our immunity and communicate with our body on a level so intricate it can change our genetic destiny.

Integrative Medicine

If you suspect you have intestinal hyperpermeability and visit a doctor about it, how will he or she address the problem? Chapter 4 laid out the details of some baseline diagnostic tests that integrative practitioners might suggest. Here, we give an overview of how integrative medicine approaches leaky gut.

CAM and integrative professionals tend to use a broader panel of diagnostic tests than conventional practitioners and use this data in conjunction with anecdotal evidence from the patient's account of his or her experiences and symptoms. All of these factors are taken into account when devising comprehensive treatment strategies that address the body and the mind of a leaky gut patient.

Integrative Medicine and Diagnostics

Some common causes of leaky gut can be determined by laboratory tests for specific intestinal infections (like candida and other SIBO), food allergies, abnormal levels of pancreatic enzymes, and toxic chemicals. If candida is the culprit, drugs like Nystatin, Nizoral, and Diflucan can be prescribed while the patient is instructed to avoid the sugars and simple carbohydrates in which candida thrive. If the cause was trauma or the long-term use of NSAIDs like naproxen, ibuprofen, or aspirin, the protocol will likely include specific dietary guidelines and probiotics to heal the intestinal lining.

GUT WISE

The bacteria in your gut can detect your stress levels. During and after a traumatic event like an accident, a death in the family, or losing a job, your brain produces hormones that can cause normally healthy gut bacteria to mutate into pathogenic strains. This is another important reason to manage your stress and develop healthy coping mechanisms and strong social and family bonds that can ease you through stressful times. It's good for the mind, body, soul, and gut bacteria.

Another specific test that dietitians and other CAM professionals employ to diagnose leaky gut is the lactulose/mannitol test. To prepare for this lab, you fast for 8 hours (or simply overnight) and provide a baseline morning urine sample from home. At the testing site, you drink a mixture of lactulose and mannitol, which are two different kinds of sugars that under normal circumstances, mostly remain in your GI tract after digestion.

Your levels lactulose/mannitol levels are then tested repeatedly in urine samples collected over the next 6 hours. If you have a high count of these sugars, then your intestine is most likely hyperpermeable. This test, while not perfect, can help patients see progress over time because as their intestinal barrier function improves, the lactulose/mannitol ratio in their urine should reflect that improvement.

A holistic approach is best when treating a leaky gut. Although the diagnostics tests are varied and improving all the time, none of them are 100 percent conclusive. Dr. Alessio Fasano, the discoverer of zonulin, is currently hard at work on fail-safe diagnostic tools for intestinal hyper-permeability. In the meantime, the best preventative action we can take is to eat healthy foods rich in nutrients; avoid gluten, which increases the production of zonulin in everyone; and exercise regularly.

Integrative Medicine and the Body and Mind Prescriptions

Specific dietary protocols for leaky gut will vary from patient to patient according to their prior lifestyle and eating habits, their symptoms, and their test results. The dietary protocols tend to start out very restrictive in order to determine which foods, if any, cause reactions or irritation. These eliminations also give the gut lining a break and give it a chance to heal. Gradually, patients reintroduce foods into the diet to see how well they're tolerated. The dietary prescription usually involves most, if not all, of the following recommendations:

- Food sensitivities must be identified by eliminating the most common allergens: wheat, dairy, refined sugar, corn, soy, eggs, peanuts, citrus fruits, chocolate, and fermented products. (See Chapter 8 for more on elimination diets.)

- Avoid fried foods, spicy foods, alcohol, and caffeine.

- Drink plenty of water to aid in detoxing the body.

- Eat fresh leafy green and cruciferous vegetables, fish, organic free-range chicken, and quinoa or small portions of whole-grain brown rice.

- Take prescribed supplements that encourage beneficial bacterial growth (such as zinc, magnesium, vitamin A, probiotics, and herbals like grapeseed extract).

Integrative medicine also takes stock of the emotional and even spiritual well-being of the patient. The brain-gut axis is real, and stress management is an integral part of getting intestinal hyperpermeability under control. Bodywork like acupuncture, massage therapy, and chiropractic adjustments can help keep inflammation and stress levels in check. These treatments also improve circulation and aid in detoxification. Mind-body practices such as yoga, tai-chi, and qi gong can build muscle and strength and calm an overtaxed nervous system.

GUT WISE

In addition to being a great stress reliever, yoga directly contributes to a healthy gut. Twisting while seated or standing helps manage and reduce gas and bloating and promotes regularity. Bending forward and holding that pose compresses your abdominal organs, but when you right yourself fresh blood and oxygen flood your GI tract, giving it a boost.

When problems arise as a result of leaky gut, we can work toward a diagnosis by working with integrative practitioners to determine how our symptoms correlate to diet and work to heal the gut from there. We examine how to do this, primarily through diet, in Part 4. Additionally, in Parts 4 and 5, we address some of the more specific dietary protocols CAM and integrative medical professionals might prescribe and oversee.

The Least You Need to Know

- Intestinal hyperpermeability occurs when zonulin widens the spaces between cells in the gut lining, allowing antigens into the circulatory system.

- Leaky gut increases your body's exposure to antigens, increasing the chances of your bad genes being activated.

- Nutrition can influence our health at the genetic level.

- Gut bacteria play a role in communicating with our DNA, so make choices that aid in keeping gut populations in balance.

- Epigenetics is proving that gut health has an influence on which genes are activated in our body.

- It's important to be proactive about your health and seek out a more integrative medical team who stays on top of the most current advances in gut health.

CHAPTER 6

Problems with the Typical Diet

A lot of people cringe when they hear "healthy diet" or "healthy" anything. Sometimes we're programmed to associate these concepts with sacrifice. We don't want to give up what tastes good and what makes us feel satisfied and comforted. While there is certainly pleasure to be derived from eating unhealthy foods, there are many more pleasures in having lots of energy, an outstanding immune system, and optimal gut health.

In this chapter, we examine how the typical diet undermines our gut health goals. When our diet is stacked with the wrong kind of calories, we set ourselves up for digestive problems that spread to other systems in the body. Processed foods, in particular, are the nemesis of good health. They're chock-full of substances that taste good, but this is a fleeting pleasure. When we understand the impact of common triggers with processed foods, it becomes easier to focus on the reward of good health. We can claim the energy and well-being that comes from healing the gut and working in symbiosis with your microbiota to feel your best and mitigate, reverse, and prevent disease.

In This Chapter

- The negative gut health impacts of consuming empty calories
- The dangers of excess salt and refined sugars
- Common food allergens and why they trigger gut problems
- What processed foods do to your gut

How the Typical Diet Affects the Body

The typical diet is comprised of too many sugars, the wrong kinds of carbs and salts, too little fiber, and too many empty calories we don't burn off. The effects these bad habits have on the digestive system are disastrous. They range from irregularity, uncomfortable gas, and acid reflux to autoimmune disorders, diabetes, learning disabilities, and heart disease.

One of the major issues plaguing the typical diet is processed and denatured food products that have been stripped of their original nutrients and then replaced with salt and refined sugars. Repeated exposure to excess salts and sugar actually desensitize your taste buds over time and makes it necessary for you to up the sugar and salt content for there to be any "taste" to food. These artificially boosted flavors distort your taste buds and sensory receptors in your brain. In short, you can get addicted to how the food products taste and how they make you feel.

 YOU ARE WHAT YOU EAT

Virgin coconut oil is a healthy saturated fat to use at room temperature or in cooking. Coconut oil is 50 percent lauric acid, one of the components in human breast milk. After we ingest coconut oil or any form of lauric acid, the body converts it into mono-laurin, which fights fungi, pathogenic bacteria, and viruses. So let the coconut oil flow. Your gut bacteria, and your body as a whole, will thank you.

The good news is that once you remove excess sugar and salt from your diet, if you're patient, healthy food will taste better to you. You will get satisfaction from a salad and be turned off by artificial flavors. This taste bud transformation solves the other problems inherent in the typical diet. If you can wean yourself off the excess sugars and salt, especially in processed foods, you can avoid the pitfalls of a warped metabolism, enjoy foods with natural fiber your digestive system loves, and consume the right kind of calories for a healthy gut.

The Wrong Kind of Calories

"But consuming the wrong kind of calories feels so good!" This is the complaint we can almost hear from people reluctant to change. And they have a reason to whine. The typical diet is loaded with sugars, carbs, and the kind of fats that combine to form quite a "feel-good cocktail" in our body. Be advised—the high doesn't last forever, and it doesn't come without a price.

Sugar, carbs, and fat can actually mitigate the effects of stress because they increase *endorphin* and *dopamine* levels in our brains. They release other neurotransmitters like *serotonin* that make us feel as if everything in life is just fine and dandy. There is a danger to eating foods overloaded with sugars, simple carbohydrates, and processed fats, especially during times of stress.

> **DEFINITION**
>
> **Endorphins** are proteins produced by your central nervous system that act like natural opiates. Your body releases them during stress and pain to reduce your discomfort. **Dopamine** acts as both a neurotransmitter and a hormone. It plays a role in regulating your mood. **Serotonin** is a neurotransmitter produced in the brain and intestine and plays a role in our mood and pain perception.

When you eat the wrong kind of calories during times of stress, you end up programming your brain to continue those bad habits. The combination of pleasure hormones rushing through your system in response to both the unhealthy foods *and* the stress hormones can cause adaptations in your nerve pathways to want to repeat that behavior. Additionally, studies have shown that food reward and sensitivity is decreased during stress. In other words, when you're really stressed out you don't actually enjoy the food that you're eating as much as you do when you're calmer. And so you keep eating because you're not getting the food reward you're expecting. It's just like an addict who develops a tolerance for a drug and has to take a bigger and bigger dose to feel a high.

It would be nice if the high also delivered a nutritional punch, but sadly, it doesn't. The calories in the typical diet offer little nutritional payoff. On average, Americans in particular receive less than 5 percent of their calories from unrefined plant foods high in nutrients. This dietary imbalance leaves a person vulnerable to deficiencies and unable to produce key enzymes needed for basic cell functions. It spells disaster for gut health in general. A lack of plant-based nutrients can weaken the immune system and contribute to pathogenic bacteria overgrowth in the gut microbiome, such as small intestinal bacterial overgrowth (SIBO).

Another contributing factor to wrong calorie consumption is the medical community demonizing the wrong fats for more than 50 years. For half a century, saturated fats, in general, were lumped into the "unhealthy" category, and a large number of people and food manufacturers heeded this advice. The result was the dawn of the man-made alternative—*trans fats*. We now understand to be a major threat to gut health and general well-being.

> **DEFINITION**
>
> **Trans fats** are also called trans fatty acids. They are man-made compounds produced by using heavy metals to get hydrogen atoms to bind to vegetable oils. They raise cholesterol levels and cause other damage to the body.

Trans fats, made up mostly of hydrogenated vegetable oils, were hailed as a healthier alternative to natural animal fats and saturated vegetable-based fats such as palm and coconut oils. Worse yet, in an effort to make food "low-fat" in general, refined sugars were often added to foods to boost flavor. This was a recipe for consuming the wrong kind of calories that promote disease, gut bacteria imbalance, and compromised immune function.

The Dangers of High Energy Intake and Low Energy Output

Modern life affords us the ability to spend time enjoying intellectual, spiritual, and leisurely pursuits while our ancestors had to devote their lives to hunting and gathering. A side effect of modern life for many people is an expanding waistline. This is a result of consuming too many of the wrong calories and then not using those calories. Most of us aren't burning off calories by foraging in the woods or chasing animals all day. A calorie is a unit of energy contained in food, and our cells convert the nutrients in food into usable energy for cell function. But what happens if you've consumed too much energy?

Your body will store any extra calories you consume in lean tissue and fat cells, but mostly in fat cells. You put pressure on all the systems of your body if you engage in high energy intake and low energy output. Your pancreas has to work overtime pumping out insulin to convert extra sugar into usable energy. The presence of all that insulin sends signals to the body to store more fat because there's already plenty of usable energy in the system. Your pancreas doesn't know that you don't plan on burning it off. It's another vicious cycle. The more empty calories you eat, the more blood sugar spikes, the more your body is programmed to store fat.

> **GUT WISE**
>
> The link between diet and disease is often very direct. In rural China, less than 1 percent of women develop breast cancer, but in America where women over-whelmingly consume a "typical diet" the statistic is 18 percent. When Asian women immigrate to America where more processed choices abound, they suffer the same rates as American women.

If you're overeating and not getting up and moving around, you're making life very hard for your gut. Sedentary lifestyles increase transit time in your intestine. This can lead to irritable bowel syndrome (IBS), constipation, and painful gas caused by food fermenting in your gut because, like you, it's staying still for too long. Have you ever heard the saying, "a rolling stone gathers no moss"? Well, a moving gut gathers no pathogens. The longer you sit still and keep consuming calories you don't use, the longer food sits and festers in your gut. This is just the opportunity the bad bacteria pounce on to get out of control and binge themselves on whatever sugars and simple carbs you've laid out for them to eat. Laying out the pathogen banquet on a regular basis leads to enterocyte degeneration, gut dysbiosis (microbiota imbalance), and gut hyperpermeability.

Lack of Fiber and the Lower GI Tract

There are so many healthy substances lacking in the typical diet, and we can add fiber to that list. The American Dietetic Association recommends that people consume between 20 and 30 grams of fiber a day. So what is fiber exactly, and why is it important to gut health?

Fiber is a carbohydrate but with some important distinctions. Fiber is different from other carbs, proteins, and fats because your body doesn't digest it. But it does need it. Dietary fiber refers to the bits of plant matter we don't actually absorb. There are two types of fiber, and they benefit our bodies in distinct ways. Soluble fiber dissolves in water and is known to lower cholesterol and blood sugar. You can find it in beans, peas, oats, apples, carrot, barley, citrus fruits, and psyllium. Insoluble fiber doesn't dissolve, so it moves through your digestive system relatively intact and promotes healthy stool formation. You can find it in nuts, beans, most vegetables, and whole wheat.

GUT WISE

Fiber supplements can be helpful to gut health if you use them properly and understand which type of fiber you're choosing to get the results you need. Supplementing with small to moderate amounts of soluble fibers, known as prebiotics, are like food for the gut flora and help regulate bowel movements. However, supplementing with insoluble fiber can be irritating to our guts. Be "gut wise" when choosing a fiber supplement.

We discuss some issues with beans and wheat later in this chapter, but for now know that consuming a wide variety of insoluble and soluble fiber is important to digestive health. The problem with the typical diet is that it provides too little of the right kind of fiber. Dietary fiber softens stools and makes them easier to pass. Bowel movements that have the heft and weight of fiber lower the risk of hemorrhoids and *diverticulitis*. Soluble fiber has the capacity to slow sugar absorption and regulate blood sugar to help mitigate diabetes or reduce the risk of developing the disease. Fiber ferments in the lower portion of your GI tract and produces short-chain fatty acids, which may prevent colorectal cancer. We need this powerful substance to keep our digestive tract running smoothly.

Sodium: A Balancing Act

Like fat, sodium has been demonized in the medical field, and while there are good reasons for that, we need to make some important distinctions. Not all sodium is created equal. Crystal salt and the sea salt that occur in nature are much different from the sodium chloride manufactured for industrial use and the sodium chloride commonly labeled as "table salt."

Naturally occurring salts contain sodium chloride, but this compound is paired with trace minerals already found in the human body. When sodium chloride is consumed without these mineral in tow, the compound pulls water into itself and causes water retention in the body, high blood pressure, and circulation troubles. It puts pressure on the body to deal with the excess sodium, and the extra processes that attempt to handle the excess often lead to gallstones and kidney stones.

> **YOU ARE WHAT YOU EAT**
>
> Commercially produced iodized table salt is not paired with micronutrients that help our bodies absorb and use it properly. In its natural state, salt contains only small amounts of iodine, but it has other micronutrients that help iodine get absorbed more efficiently. When looking for a table salt alternative, steer clear of anything labeled "refined." Look for sea salts with a mineral-rich appearance and texture. Let your eyes be the judge, and follow your gut!

In nature, sodium chloride is found in deposits alongside trace elements such as potassium, zinc, magnesium, and calcium. Sodium chloride consumed in isolation from these trace minerals causes those same elements in our own body to be thrown out of balance. A fear of consuming too much sodium chloride does not mean we should avoid salt. It means we need to be mindful of the source of the salt and use it in moderation.

We need salt in our diets just as much as we need water. Sodium chloride is an *electrolyte* crucial to basic cell function. Most electrolytes help regulate the balance of fluids outside our bodies' cells with fluids inside of cells. They help our body systems achieve homeostasis. We need electrolytes to conduct the messages in our nervous systems, to help us to stay hydrated, and to enable muscle function. Sodium chloride is an important electrolyte, but it needs to be in balance with the body's needs.

> **DEFINITION**
>
> **Diverticulitis** is the inflammation of small pouches that line the wall of the colon. **Electrolytes** are substances that split into their separate ions in a solution and are capable of conducting electricity. Salt (sodium chloride) splits into its separate components in water and in the body helps conduct nerve impulses and aids in homeostasis.

Research dating back to the 1970s shows that diets high in sodium chloride (table salt) increase the risk for heart attack and heart disease in general. Too much table salt weakens blood vessels and leads to high blood pressure. New studies also indicate that too much sodium in the diet can promote the production of too many T-cells (white blood cells that attack foreign invaders). This increase in white blood cells can cause widespread inflammation in the body and lead to autoimmunity. If a person is already suffering from leaky gut and some genetic markers for auto-immune disease, too much table salt can have disastrous consequences.

While excess salt in the body is expelled through urine, it takes other crucial minerals along with it like calcium and magnesium. Over time, this can lead to osteoporosis. Just another reason why salt intake is a delicate balance in which to be aware.

The U.S. Department of Agriculture (USDA) currently recommends 2,300 milligrams of sodium a day, but even that might be too much. Keeping your intake between 1,000 and 2,000 milligrams is a safe bet for good health. Helpful habits to help you regulate sodium are eating whole foods and avoiding processed food that add loads of table salt that desensitize your taste buds. As you decrease your sodium intake, you will learn to appreciate the natural sodium that occurs in almost all foods. You might not have noticed their natural brininess when your taste buds were on overdrive from the added table salt.

The instinct you might have after hearing about the dangers of table salt is to cut sodium chloride out of your diet altogether. As you phase out processed foods and increase your intake of whole foods high in nutrients, you will take in enough sodium and be able to trust your natural ability to detect "saltiness." If you still feel like you'd like a little more, don't despair. Remember, not all salt is created equal. Salt your foods with Celtic sea salt or Himalayan salt, which contain other beneficial minerals as well. It's the processed sodium chloride that needs to stay off limits.

Inflammation, Immune Responses, and Allergens: Major Food Triggers

Allergies are immune responses to an irritant that enters our system. Our immune system starts producing antibodies to fight the perceived invader and inflammation is often the result. Now more than ever, food allergies are on the rise, and a lot of people want to know why. As with everything else we've discussed, the answers lie in our guts. When our gut microbiome is thrown out of whack, so is the 70 to 80 percent of our immune system that lives there. A deranged immune system will attack healthy tissues and build antibodies against proteins we once enjoyed, such as those in our favorite foods. Inflammation and a damaged gut lining results. Eat. React. Inflame. Repeat.

The modern chemical agents we use to disinfect our bodies and our homes only contribute to the problem because they deprive us of the opportunity to build up immunity to allergens we don't ingest, such as dust or pollen. Being overly hygienic also hurts the diversity of our microbiome. Frequent doses of antibiotics to fight off common infections further compromise the balance of gut microbiota. Pathogenic microbes contribute to a damaged and hyperpermeable intestinal wall that lets even more undigested foods into the bloodstream for round after round of antigen exposure, over-reactive immune responses, even more food intolerances or allergies, and even more overgrowth of pathogenic microbes.

Pathogenic bacteria can damage our immune cells' ability to properly fight infections. They can also lead to overproduction of the immune cells that travel the fluids of the body and gather at infection and injury sites to destroy invaders. Too many of these cells can cause inflammation.

Immunoglobulin E (IgE) is one type of immune cell that can go into overdrive during leaky gut, and IgE is the master of allergic responses. Let's examine five of the most common food triggers involved in this cycle.

Gluten

Dr. Fasano's research has concluded that beyond celiac disease, a much larger percentage of the public suffers from gluten sensitivity than we previously thought. No doubt, more people have actively investigated their long-standing "mystery symptoms" in recent years, especially with the advent of gluten-free products and increased awareness about celiac and gluten intolerance. So what happens in people whose bodies treat gluten like an invader?

The skin of your intestine (the serosa) is very wrinkled and folded. If you were to take it out of your body and lay it out, it would be the size of a tennis court. The inside of the cavity that forms the tube of your intestine is called the lumen, and this houses all of the bacteria that lie within the gut.

Gluten is not a problem if it stays within the tube of the lumen, because then it ends up in the toilet where it should. But this does not happen for people with celiac disease, those predisposed to autoimmune disorders, and those whose bacteria population is imbalanced. In these folks, the gluten is not broken down properly. Instead, it makes its way into the bloodstream. As long as these people eat gluten, the body acts as if it is under a never-ending attack.

ASK THE EXPERTS

Dr. Alessio Fasano has suggested that if infants avoid gluten during their first year, they are four times less likely to develop celiac disease. Perhaps it's time to rethink the conventional protocol of introducing grains to infants as their first solid foods. Talk with an integrative practitioner experienced in pediatric nutrition to discuss alternatives to this protocol, especially if you have a family history of autoimmune disorders.

According to Dr. Fasano, people can develop an intolerance for gluten at any age. So what flips the on-switch for intolerance? The genes for an autoimmune reaction lay dormant until changes in the microbiome causes their communication between our immune system and intestinal wall to go haywire. And these changes are brought about by unhealthy, processed food.

Dr. Fasano's and his team of scientists conducted a study of 3,000 adults over the course of 30 years. They wanted to see how many of them developed celiac disease and what happened in their lives that may have been an influencing factor. What they discovered was that between the 1970s and 2000 the rate of celiac disease more than quadrupled. It went from 1 in 500 people in the 1970s to 1 in 100 in the year 2000.

Among the subjects of the study were two women who didn't develop an intolerance to gluten until their late 70s. Dr. Fasano concluded that the most probable cause for these women's spontaneous autoimmune response to gluten, after more than 70 years of consuming it, was gut bacteria. He also concluded that this spike in the onset of celiac disease in the general population over the past 40 years is due to drastic changes in the human microbiome. These changes can happen from antibiotic use and from an increase in processed food consumption. These changes are drastic enough to stimulate the expression of genes for gluten-induced autoimmunity at any age.

Grains

Many grains beside wheat also contain gluten, which cause the production of zonulin that leads to open tight junctions and an overly porous intestinal wall. Undigested grains running rampant in our circulatory system cause inflammation and immune dysfunction, which in a lot of cases, manifests as a food allergy.

Unprocessed whole grains are effective at curbing our appetite and making us feel satisfied, but the fact is they don't contain enough micronutrients to form a huge block of our diets. The trouble is, for most people, processed grains like white flour make up a huge portion of the calories they consume every day. These refined carbohydrates have been linked to obesity, diabetes, heart disease, and prostate enlargement. Whole-wheat bread actually raises your blood sugar just as much as refined white table sugar does.

Refined grains also disrupt the balance of your gut homeostasis because they are a favorite food of pathogenic bacteria. They also weaken the white blood cells produced in the intestine. In this way, consuming refined grains as a large portion of your diet would contribute to the weakening of the immune system as a whole and the inflammation of the intestinal wall.

 YOU ARE WHAT YOU EAT

> Whole grains are a healthier alternative to refined grains and flours for people whose gut lining can tolerate them. However, they're less nutrient-dense and have less disease-fighting power than other members of the seed family such as chia, hemp, flax, and sesame. Try whole grains with less negative impact and more nutritional value like quinoa, oats, buckwheat, and wild rice.

Grains behave like an allergen for people with damaged intestinal walls because their enterocytes can't process certain proteins. One of the enzymes the intestinal enterocytes should produce breaks down the protein in gluten. When the intestinal wall is compromised, this protein either breaks down grains improperly or not at all.

Legumes

Legumes are high in fiber, protein, and carbohydrates. But they can be problematic for some of us, causing inflammation and acting as an allergen. The reasons lie in the biology and chemical makeup of the legumes themselves. When we eat legumes (beans, lentils, chickpeas, peanuts, etc.), we eat the seed of the plant containing all of its genetic information. The biological drive of living things is to reproduce. A seed is designed to be resilient, to be able to be eaten by animal and "deposited" into the soil after passing through an animal's gut. And we're no different. Legumes are not designed to be digested and absorbed.

Legumes also contain lectins that can cause inflammation in some people. Lectins can be found in all plants and are mostly used as defenses against pests and microorganisms, like mold. They're a kind of protein, and they're not all harmful. In fact, some research suggests that lectins are largely broken down by soaking and cooking legumes, so they don't cause problems if you have great gut microbiota and an intact gut. However, seeds will tax even a healthy digestive system because the GI tract has to work overtime to produce the enzymes needed to break them down, using up vital nutrients in the process. We get some nutrients from legumes, but the trade-off isn't outstanding. The nutritional payoff of eating legumes doesn't come close to those of other protein sources.

> **GUT WISE**
>
> The peanut is a problematic legume. In those with peanut allergies, the immune system begins an alarming response as soon as they make contact with peanuts.. Between 1997 and 2010 the rate of peanut allergies among children in the United States tripled! The exact cause of this sharp increase has yet to be determined. It would not surprise us if there is a connection to gut dysbiosis and intestinal hyperpermeability, as together these two root causes undermine the normal immune functions that prevent allergic response.

Legumes are incompletely digested under even the best of circumstances, and if your gut lining is already overly leaky, then these bits of food cause harmful immune responses, such as inflammation. *Phytates* are natural substances found in many legumes and grains that also disrupt the gut. They bind to essential minerals in our digestive system and prevent our intestinal wall from absorbing them. Phytates hinder our ability to absorb calcium, magnesium, iron, zinc, and iodide. The iodide malabsorption is especially problematic in children because iodide plays a key role in thyroid function, which helps regulate the growing process and brain development.

Legumes are also hard on our guts because they're high in "difficult to digest" *FODMAPs,* which is an acronym for fermentable oligosaccharides, disaccharides, monosaccharides, and polyols. There are many foods with high FODMAPs content, and legumes are on the short list of biggest offenders. Here's why FODMAPs are a problem: they aren't easily absorbed in the small intestine. If they just sit there, they become food for the pathogenic bacteria whose by-products give you uncomfortable bloating and even diarrhea. Because they're such great food for bacteria, legumes can also lead to SIBO. Yet another contributor to the gut dysbiosis that leads us down the path to increased intestinal hyperpermeability and immune dysfunction. (We have more on FODMAPs in Chapter 10.)

If you already have other food allergies, sensitivities, and/or symptoms of intestinal hyperpermeability, lay off the legumes until your gut has healed. Even then, eat them in small quantities. They're certainly tasty and have some nutritional value, but there are too many solid reasons why legumes should not be the primary source of protein in your diet.

Dairy

Milk is controversial when it comes to maintaining gut health. Whether or not you can tolerate dairy varies according to both your genetics and your gut microbes. In people with abnormal gut microbiota and therefore intestinal hyperpermeability, dairy can cause a lot of problems. Although your predisposition for lactose intolerance is an inherited trait, you're more likely to have the problem if you're of African, Asian, or Mediterranean descent.

When we eat dairy, digestive juices in the stomach split milk proteins into amino acids. Normally these amino acids should be sent along to the small intestine to be further broken down by the microvilli of the cells of the gut wall but that step only happens if the person's microbiota are balanced and working properly to help nutrient absorption. When we suffer gut dysbiosis, the amino acids aren't broken down. They get sent into the circulatory system unchanged.

The same amino acid process happens for gluten with the same incomplete breakdown for those with gut dysbiosis and hyperpermeable intestinal walls. If the integrity of your intestinal walls is compromised, eating gluten or dairy allows antigens to roam the body and the immune system launches an attack, causing inflammation and even autoimmunity.

In some cases, people with dairy allergies lack the enzyme lactase, which allows us to properly digest *lactose*, the sugar in milk. In fact, about 70 percent of people worldwide have some level of lactose intolerance that prevents them from fully digesting the milk sugar. Undigested lactose ferments in the intestine and leads to uncomfortable gas, bloating, and even diarrhea. Those other 30 percent are the lucky people with healthy gut bacteria populations have just the right amount of E. coli bacteria, which do the job of breaking down the lactose in milk.

When the gut population is balanced and diverse, digesting dairy isn't a problem. In addition to it acting as an allergen for many people, especially for those with compromised gut health, casein, the protein in dairy, has been shown to elevate IGF-1 levels in the blood. IGF-1 is a substance much like insulin. It stimulates cell growth, but unfortunately some studies show that it also promotes the growth of abnormal cells like cancer cells. This happens much more often with low-fat milk options that have been highly processed.

> **DEFINITION**
>
> **Phytates** are compounds in legumes and grains that bind to essential minerals, making it difficult for the enterocytes to absorb them. **FODMAPs** is the acronym for fermentable oligosaccharides, disaccharides, monosaccharides, and polyols. These substances are hard for the small intestine to digest, and in susceptible individuals they can feed pathogenic bacteria. **Lactose** is the naturally occurring sugar in milk.

So what should you do about dairy? If you notice that dairy consumption coincides with unpleasant skin, bowel, bloating, or breathing issues, then phase it out of your diet. You can always try to introduce it after several weeks, or even months. We recommend some dairy guidelines in Parts 4 and 5. You may not have to give up dairy permanently, and there's good reason to embrace certain types of dairy products. The calcium in dairy products can be absorbed by the body more easily than most vegetable sources of calcium.

If dairy is consumed, the recommendation by a lot of nutrition experts is that it be from a trusted source where you can consume it raw (if available and approved in your area), full-fat, and organic. Better yet is fermented dairy like yogurt or kefir that feed your beneficial microbiota with naturally occurring probiotics.

Sugar

It is ingrained into our DNA to like sweet foods over savory because foods that taste sweet in the wild most likely will not kill you. We also evolved to have color vision and be attracted to the bright colors of ripe fruit. These mechanisms train our brains to think, "Yay! This won't kill me." Unfortunately processed foods manufacturers utilize these instincts to lead us to sugary foods instead of fruit.

Fruit is full of micronutrients. Refined sugar, however, will destroy your gut microbiota population, leading to inflammation and other problems. We should be very concerned about the effects of refined sugar on the body, as the average Western person consumes around 160 pounds of the stuff every year.

YOU ARE WHAT YOU EAT

Frozen fruit is comparable in nutritional value to fresh fruit. When something is out of season, especially in winter months, don't skimp on fruit consumption, simply opt for frozen options. Canned fruits usually contain added sweeteners or are cooked before they're canned and lose a lot of their nutritional punch.

There are different forms of sugar, and just like salts, they are not all created equally. Your body just processes them differently. Here's the rundown of the two major types of sugar:

Monosaccharides: Include glucose and fructose, which are found in fruits, vegetables, and even honey; and galactose, which is found in dairy, legumes, and some fruits and vegetables. Monosaccharides are easily digested and absorbed by enterocytes in most cases.

Disaccharides: Include sucrose, which is the main component of white table sugar and natural sources like maple syrup; lactose, which is the sugar in milk; and maltose, the sugar from starch digestion. Disaccharides take more work than monosaccharides to break down. If someone already has a compromised gut lining, then their enterocytes won't make the enzymes needed to break down these larger sugars. In people with leaky guts, disaccharides stay in the gut and feed pathogenic bacteria, setting off more negative chain reactions.

One of the most common imbalances resulting from too much sugar in the digestive tract is an overgrowth of candida and clostridia. These two pathogens, and the toxins they produce, impair the enterocytes' ability to further break down the complex carbohydrates in grains and starchy vegetables. This becomes another vicious cycle contributing to gut dysbiosis because those undigested carbs feed more pathogenic bacteria instead of nourishing you. Whatever undigested carbs the pathogens don't eat ferments in the intestine and further contributes to gut mucosa damage and immune system problems. All of these factors also exacerbate leaky gut, inflammation, and other disastrous health consequences over time.

Refined sugar has really caused an epidemic of gut-related problems in the modern world. Fructose in fruit used to be the main source of sugar in the human body. Sugar cane has been cultivated in many countries for millennia, but until the seventeenth century it was a considered a fine spice and not a staple ingredient. As manufacturing processes improved in the nineteenth and twentieth centuries, sugar became cheaper and more commonly used. Then, in 1975, high fructose corn was invented and hit the supermarket shelves in processed foods and made its way into our lives. It's incredibly cheap to produce, and incredibly dangerous to gut health.

The bottom line is that we're all eating too much sugar and simple carbs that turn into sugar. Fat consumption is down from 20 years ago, but sugar consumption from soda and fruit cocktails has skyrocketed. These sugars cause gut dysbiosis by contributing specifically to candida overgrowth and SIBO.

A Closer Look at Processed Food

Processing depletes natural foods of their nutrients and chemically alters them to increase their shelf life and artificially boost flavor. Here's the really insidious thing about processed foods: their manufacturers have calculated how to make them addictive. They are comprised of the right combinations of salt, sugar, and fatty textures our mouths love. Processed food producers have deliberately manipulated our flavor preferences that stoke pleasure sensors in the brain. Once we start eating them, we want to continue eating because it literally *feels* good.

The good news is that these preferences in our brains for those prepackaged and largely artificial flavors are not set in stone. We can change our preferences and how our brains are wired to interpret these flavors. But it takes time and patience. Flavor preferences are learned responses.

And as the awareness of the dangers of process foods grows, consumers are demanding more information and transparency about the inherent risks of eating these foods. Many processed food companies face impending class action lawsuits in response to their deliberate manipulation of sugar, salt, and fat ratios that have been designed to override disciplined responses in the human brain. Also in the works is legal backlash for marketing unhealthy processed foods to young children. There is even talk in the U.S. Food and Drug Administration (FDA) of assigning a daily value to sugar so nutrition labels reflect those percentages.

Refined Sugar

Processed foods are high in white refined sugars and simple carbs, and therefore have a high glycemic index (a measurement on a scale of 1 to 100 that scores the effect a food has on blood sugar levels). Carbs that occur naturally are absorbed by our body as glucose. This sugar is digested slowly and raises blood sugars levels gradually at a rate we can handle. But processed carbs are digested and absorbed quickly, and it throws our system into a taxing overdrive mode that struggles to keep up with the sugar spike and pumps out too much insulin to compensate. So about an hour later, the abundance of insulin in the system makes the person crave more sugar. Another vicious cycle to add to our growing list.

Combine their impact on blood sugar with the high fat and low nutrients of the processed fats and oils, and processed foods set up consumers for major health problems. The human body cannot properly absorb and convert these foods into energy. Fats, sugars, and carbs in their natural state are much easier for our systems to handle. Overly processed saturated and trans fats coupled with a low-nutrient diet are a recipe for disaster. The icing on this bittersweet, processed cake is the damage refined sugars and carbs do to the white blood cells produced in the gut. Frankly put, processed foods destroy our immune system.

Trans Fats

The health crisis spawned by the reign of processed foods is so dire that it has even incited government interventions. Recently the American government announced a phase-out of trans fats in foods by 2018. Trans fats were introduced into the American food supply in 1911 as a shortening used in baked goods. Margarine and other partially hydrogenated oils are now a staple in processed foods.

Most sources of trans fats are chemically engineered substances designed to be similar to animal-based saturated fats. They're cheaper than animal fats, which is what made them attractive to manufacturers of processed food. There are only small amounts of naturally occurring trans fats in dairy and in lamb, deer, and cow meat. These are chemically different from industrially created trans fats and are fine for the human body in moderation.

Man-made trans fats are created by taking an unsaturated fat, which is liquid or soft at room temperature, and adding hydrogen to the structure to mimic a saturated fat that hardens the substance. Companies do this to improve mouthfeel and extend the shelf life of a product. Over the years, companies have profited from trans fats. The health costs, however, are high.

Heating vegetable oils and binding more hydrogen atoms to them turns liquid oils into solids, which are easier to manipulate in manufactured food products. In order to get the hydrogen to fuse to the oil, heavy metals are used in the process. New research demonstrates that these residual metals in the oils can wreak havoc on the intestinal lining. The other danger to gut health is the structure of these fats. Trans fats are similar enough to the essential fats we *really* need that they trick the body into accepting them. It's kind of like forging a medical degree and then walking into an operating room. You're not going to be able to perform the job. And neither can the trans fats. These imposters interrupt the immune system, hormone production, insulin response to blood sugar, and enzyme activity.

ASK THE EXPERTS

For the first time in human history, we are witnessing overweight people who are starving. We are programmed to find the most calories with the least effort. In the natural environment where processed foods never existed, calories came in tandem with nutrients; one led us to the other. In our present environment, this more than likely is not the case. Foods have been stripped of their micronutrients, delivering instead an inordinate amount of artificially concentrated calories. It is rather easy to become simultaneously fat and malnourished.

—Mark Houliff, PhD, CNC, FAAIM, DCCN, Consultative Health and Nutrition

Trans fats are linked to increased rates of heart disease and cancer. In fact, the damage trans fats cause to the circulatory system over time can be life-threatening. One the most dangerous qualities of trans fats concerning gut health is that they are easily absorbed by the enterocytes of the intestinal wall. If you already have a leaky gut, trans fat is even more readily available to body systems and can cause an overactive immune system. How do they do this? Trans fats literally change the structure of fatty acids in our cells and make cells dysfunctional.

Acrylamides and GMOs

Another hidden danger in processed foods is the cancer-causing compounds called acrylamides that form in overcooked grains and potatoes. Potatoes and grains are some of the main ingredients in processed foods. Processed cheese, French fries, breakfast cereals, potato chips, and meats from fast food restaurants are all notoriously high in acrylamides.

Cooking food at extremely high temperature happens frequently in the world of big food processing companies. These temperatures alter the chemical makeup of the food and makes them harder for our body to digest. The longer the food sits there, the more toxic it becomes, irritating the lining of the intestines and even causing changes in the balance of gut bacteria.

Yet another hidden danger in processed foods are their incorporation of large quantities of genetically modified organisms (GMOs). GMOs have been altered from the natural state to be more pest- and drought-resistant. The trouble with those modifications, however, is that the plant proteins that ward off pests (lectins) can cause inflammation in our guts. GMOs also don't contain as many nutrients as their untainted counterparts. GMOs also contain elevated levels of agricultural herbicides like glyphosate. This herbicide in particular has been shown to attack beneficial gut microbes.

 YOU ARE WHAT YOU EAT

Soy is a major ingredient in processed foods, and over 90 percent of soybeans in the world are genetically modified. If you already have a sensitive and leaky gut, avoid soy unless it is labeled as non-GMO and organic. Opt for fermented soy products that are nutrient dense and rich in probiotics like natto and miso.

So What Can I Eat?

The proliferation of processed foods has taken over so much of the typical diet that cutting out those foods might drastically change your eating habits. So you might be feeling a little daunted by now, thinking, "If all that stuff is horrible for me, what *can* I eat?"

The good news is there's a lot you can eat, with a whole world of delicious and nutritious fresh foods awaiting you.

> **YOU ARE WHAT YOU EAT**
>
> Ditching the soda may be harder than you think, but it's a habit worth kicking. Soda manufacturers design their products to be addictive with their specific combinations of sugar, salt, and caffeine. The salt makes you thirstier. The caffeine is a diuretic, and the sugar is there to hide the salt. Soda is really no good for you at all.

We give you a comprehensive list of approved foods and examinations of dietary recommendations compiled by nutrition experts in Part 4. Some experts disagree on allowing animal products, legumes, and grains, but here's a preview of some basics.

- Eat whole foods, fruits, and vegetables.

- Gluten-free whole grains offer some fiber and nutrition but should be eaten in moderation.

- Responsibly raised (grass-fed, no antibiotics, and free-range) animal meats or fatty fish low in mercury, like salmon, are good for you in moderation.

- Fermented dairy, like yogurt, is healthy and rich in probiotics and is great for you as long as it doesn't cause you uncomfortable gas or autoimmune symptoms.

- Healthy fats can be consumed in nuts, seeds, avocados, and organic free-range eggs as long as you don't have pronounced allergic responses to them.

The key takeaways on eating for a healthy gut are moderation and patience. With that in mind, you can transition from the typical diet toward healthier eating with a commitment to outstanding health, energy, disease resistance, and the ability to overcome even bad genetics.

The Least You Need to Know

- Eating more calories than your body needs puts unnecessary stress on all of your body's systems.
- Eating too little fiber and too much sodium chloride (or table salt) raises your blood pressure and taxes your digestive and cardiovascular systems.

- Gluten, grains, dairy, and legumes contain proteins that are difficult to absorb and cause inflammation for people with leaky guts and abnormal gut bacteria.
- Refined sugar is a leading cause of health problems, from pathogenic gut bacteria overgrowth to heart disease.
- Processed foods, which are stripped of nutrients, trigger addictive eating habits and contribute to gut bacteria imbalance, leaky gut, and immune system disorders.

How Your Gut Impacts Your Health

Your gut and its microbiota interact with multiple body systems and play a crucial role in your overall health. Your digestive system manages the fuel the rest of your body needs to perform every function of every single cell. If something is awry in the digestive system, a ripple effect eventually runs the course in other areas of the body. Because the vast majority of your immune cells lie in the gut, so do the root causes of immune responses such as allergies, inflammation, and autoimmunity. Your gut also produces 95 percent of your body's serotonin, a major neurotransmitter that regulates moods. There is no doubt that the gut and its inhabitants influence our physical, emotional, and mental well-being.

In this chapter, we discuss the impact our gut has on digestion, immunity, and general physical health. We delve into the intricacies of the brain-gut axis and explain how the gut and our microbiota play a role in sensory perception and learning. We also examine how recent studies reveal connections between your gut and mental health.

In This Chapter

- An overview of digestive disorders
- How your gut microbes affect your energy levels and weight
- Links between your gut, autoimmune disorders, allergies, and respiratory problems
- Your gut and emotional health
- Learning disorders and your gut microbiome
- Gut microbiota and mental illness

Physical Health

Our gut health helps regulate our metabolism, nutrient absorption, and immune function. All of these factors contribute to the state of our physical health. If our digestive system is dysfunctional, then the quality of the energy distributed to all of our other body systems is compromised. Every cell in our body depends on the nutrients our intestine absorbs. If the lining of the gut isn't working in cooperation with the microbiome, we will feel the repercussions.

Digestion Dysfunction and Disease

In Chapter 2, we closely examined signs that your gut may be unhealthy. And in Chapter 4, we gave you a list of symptoms that warrant a trip to the doctor. In general, any long-term deviations from normal digestion that cause discomfort and interrupt your routine and quality of life is cause for a medical consultation.

> **GUT WISE**
>
> More than 40 gastrointestinal disorders can afflict our digestive systems. Upward of 34 million Americans have some form of digestive disease, and 20 million of those are chronic conditions. That means 8 percent of the U.S. population suffers with digestive diseases.

To help you track your own gut health history and symptoms, here's an overview of the seven most common dysfunctional digestive disorders and diseases:

Gastroesophageal reflux disease (GERD): Also known as persistent acid reflux, it affects 20 percent of Americans. This occurs when stomach acid flows into the esophagus due to a relaxed lower esophageal sphincter (LES) causing chest pain after a meal or when you lie down at night. While acid reflux happens to most people occasionally, if it happens twice or more a week it's considered a chronic and harmful condition that can lead to tooth and esophageal erosion, and difficulty swallowing and breathing.

Ulcers: These sores on the lining of the stomach or upper intestine can cause a lot of pain. They are caused by overactive pathogenic bacteria or abnormal GI tract secretions. If you have unexplained stomach pain, you may have one or more of these sores that can bleed internally and become infected.

Gallstones: Nearly a million American are diagnosed with these painful cholesterol and bile salt deposits every year. They cause sharp pain in the upper-right portion of your abdomen and require emergency medical treatment to avoid serious infection or rupture.

Constipation: Americans spend $725 million annually on laxatives. Constipation is a common digestive discomfort that, if chronic, leads to hemorrhoids, anal fissures, toxin accumulation, and serious colorectal problems.

Diverticulitis: This condition occurs when irregular pouches that have formed in the walls of the GI tract (most commonly in the colon) become inflamed. This inflammation can cause intense abdominal pain.

Irritable bowel syndrome (IBS): This condition is pretty much what it sounds like. Between 10 and 15 percent of Americans suffer from chronic fluctuations between constipation, diarrhea, and stomach discomfort at least three times a month for several months straight.

Inflammatory bowel disease (IBD, which includes Crohn's disease and ulcerative colitis): This condition is more serious than IBS, but often begins the same way. The symptoms persist and worsen to include rectal bleeding, anemia, weight loss, and recurring dehydration. IBD involves a malfunctioning immune system that causes chronic inflammation along the GI tract.

All seven of these afflictions have something in common. They can all be addressed by establishing a healthier gut microbiome. When these bacteria are out of balance, pathogens, along with epigenetics and other factors, lead to digestive disease.

There are other disorders of the digestive tract beyond these seven ailments. They all stem from intestinal wall irritation caused by unhealthy foods that lead to unhealthy microbiomes. Gut dysbiosis can lead to an overproduction of mucus in the gut that prevents proper digestion and nutrient absorption. All of these factors cause problems elsewhere in the body, including the brain.

Sometimes the boundaries between physical and mental health overlap, as the brain-gut axis demonstrates. We want to take some time here to discuss an overlap between physical and mental health as it concerns ulcers and IBS/IBD specifically. Remember the vagus nerve, the communication highway that creates the brain-gut axis? That's the connection that helps the brain and gut influence one another, for better or worse.

Research concludes that stress causes abnormal GI secretions and can lead to stomach ulcers. Stress, in general, can change the environment of your entire GI tract. The microbiota in your gut can also detect stress hormones and react accordingly. Psychological stress has been proven to suppress the growth of beneficial bacteria like lactobacilli and promote the growth of pathogenic E. coli.

YOU ARE WHAT YOU EAT

People with IBS should limit their fructose intake. Although fruit is healthy and full of nutrients, IBS suffers can't always absorb fructose properly, which leads to gas pains that are intolerable for them and their lower pain thresholds (caused by the increased activation of their brain's pain circuits).

Abnormal gut bacteria populations and stress also play a role in the onset and exacerbation of IBS and IBD, although there have been more conclusive studies in IBS. IBS is the result of disturbance in the gut-brain axis. In fact, more than half of IBS patients also have a psychiatric disorder. IBS patients suffer from increased activation of pain circuits in the brain, so they actually experience pain more intensely. They have a decreased pain threshold and endure a hypersensitive state that causes even normal levels of gas in the GI tract to feel unbearable.

Energy and Weight Issues

Those versatile and all-important gut microbes also impact our energy levels, metabolism, and body weight. What we eat affects the microbiota population and our microbial composition affects appetite control and nutrient absorption. The relationship is certainly a two-way street.

The lining of our gut secretes all kinds of neurotransmitters and hormones, and our microbes interact with these substances. Gut microbiota even play a role in monitoring the levels of appetite-regulating hormones. Our microbiota also help absorb nutrients and break down sugars and carbs that our bodies can't. When healthy gut population distributions are upset by unhealthy diets, these microbes no longer help us absorb nutrients properly.

Gut irritation resulting from abnormal microbiota leads to leaky gut and negative immune responses. In these instances, whatever nutrients the body is absorbing are redirected toward the energy needed to continue the immune response to antigens a leaky gut disperses into circulation. Our body will then naturally crave additional nutrients to replace what we spent on our immune response. Then, the microbiota trigger the release of more appetite hormones. This cycle is one way people become overweight.

We often consume more calories because our bodies are nutrient-starved even though we're getting plenty of fat and carbs. The fat gets stored, but there still aren't enough nutrients to fight the cycle of immune responses necessary to fight off the leaky gut attack. In turn, we feel hungry, but too often we don't feed the gut and its microbiota what they *really* need.

Nutrient-hunger is just one of four major factors affecting body-weight issues. Most weight-loss diets focus on calorie intake when they need to be focused on all four aspects involved in satiating hunger: calories, volume, nutrients, and addiction/craving. You can cut portions, but if you're not getting the nutrients your body needs to perform optimally, you'll still generate the feeling of hunger as we just discussed. "Nutrient hunger" is when the temptation to give into cravings often happens. We find ourselves taking in more calories to feel full and satisfied without taking into consideration the quality of the food.

GUT WISE

Snacking impacts your gut health by making it harder for your digestive system to produce the enzymes necessary for digestion. A digestive system really needs to rest between meals. If you're an athlete or physical laborer, you will need to snack. Most of us, however, snack more out of psychological drives than physical ones.

To deal with hunger effectively while maintaining a healthy gut, try eating a high volume of low-calorie nutrient-rich food. You won't get the big dopamine rush that comes with high-calorie foods, but over time your brain will adjust. The nutrient-dense food that cuts out processed and refined sugars and grains will also promote beneficial bacteria growth. If you are in touch with satisfying nutrition needs, unhealthy cravings will dissipate. And you can focus on eating foods that help your GI tract work in conjunction with your gut bacteria to keep your immune system strong and provide your body with energy to keep you feeling great.

Autoimmune Disorders and Diseases

Gut health is critical to maintaining immune function, and your microbiota play an important role in this. When you don't have enough healthy bacteria, the immune cells that travel to the sites of infection and inflammation and destroy viruses and toxins can no longer do their jobs. Scientists don't yet understand exactly how the bacteria help immune cell function, but they can see the results when there aren't enough beneficial bacteria. These results fluctuate wildly. Sometimes it's like an ill-equipped army fighting an enemy that drastically outnumbers them. Other times, it's like an overzealous army causing chaos by seeking and destroying both friend and foe.

One example of how overzealous immune responses get activated is in the "lines of defense" relationship between your two main types of T-cells. Your T-cell helper type 1 (Th1) cells are everywhere your body is exposed to outside influences, such as your skin and mucous membranes. Your T-cell helper type 2 (Th2) cells are deeper in the liquids of your body. Both of these immune cells rely on healthy microbiota populations to function well. When microbiota are imbalanced and abnormal, they're not communicating well with T-cells. If the Th1 cells don't do their job of providing a first line of defense, then foreign invaders penetrate the liquids of the body and Th2 soldiers, your "back-up" defenders, go into action. Over time, Th2 soldiers on constant duty attack healthy tissues, which leads to autoimmune disorders.

There are other routes to autoimmunity as well, and they also involve gut microbe populations. Poor diet and environmental factors can decimate the beneficial bacteria and let pathogenic bacteria like candida take over. Candida overgrowth can lead to toxic levels of bacterial metabolism by-products like acetaldehyde.

Acetaldehyde is dangerous because it has the ability to change the structure of proteins. Proteins are the building blocks of hormones and enzymes crucial to bodily functions. Deformed proteins can give rise to autoimmune responses that cause the body to make antibodies against itself. This leads to conditions like rheumatoid and psoriatic arthritis, in which the body attacks its own joints and skin; or multiple sclerosis, where the body attacks the lining of the cells in the brain and nervous system.

Although celiac disease affects the digestive system, it is by its very nature, an autoimmune condition, as is gluten sensitivity. Celiac is often hard to diagnose because its symptoms can be vague and mimic those of other diseases. Celiac disease can affect a lot of different organs; it can give you stomachaches, fatigue, anemia, and tingling in your fingertips. It's often hard to pinpoint, and patients often receive several misdiagnoses before the problem is identified conclusively.

Celiac disease can cause immune responses to gluten so severe they damage the villi intestinal wall. Additionally, there are many individuals who do not have celiac disease but still present with gluten sensitivity, and their immune response still causes uncomfortable inflammation both in the intestine and elsewhere in the body. In celiac disease, the gluten precipitates a rush of zonulin that leaves the tight junctions open for prolonged periods of time. Gluten sensitivity causes a similar, though less extreme, tight junction response that allows just enough gluten into the bloodstream to incite an immune response.

Skin Issues and Disorders

Your skin is an organ—your largest organ. We often neglect this fact and regard issues on our skin as purely cosmetic in nature. Skin problems, in general, are usually prompted by problems elsewhere in the body. We've discussed the brain-gut axis, but there's also a gut-skin axis as well, and the gut microbes play a role even on the outermost layer of your body.

Gut problems that can manifest as eczema, dermatitis, acne, rosacea, and other skin conditions include:

Gut dysbiosis: The imbalance of gut microbes where the pathogenic strains outnumber the probiotic ones.

Small intestinal bacterial overgrowth (SIBO): Where some strains of microbes that usually reside in the large intestine (or colon) work their way into your small intestine.

Candida overgrowth or Candidiasis: When this yeast population explodes it causes inflammation throughout your body, even your skin.

Low stomach acid: This condition compromises the digestion of carbs and leads to pathogenic overgrowths associated with acne and similar skin eruptions.

Leaky gut: The pathogens floating around your system can lead to inflammatory responses from your skin.

The gut-skin axis further illustrates the interconnectivity of the systems of your body, with your gut at the center. Your GI tract is your fuel line, and your skin is your first point of contact with the outside world. Providing healthy fuel will heal your systems from the inside out.

Inflammatory Responses and Allergies

There is no doubt that allergies are on the rise, especially food allergies. Emerging science continues to make connections explaining the epidemic of allergies and inflammatory conditions and the relationship between our food supply, our gut microbes, and how diseases and allergic reactions manifest in our bodies. There is a lot at stake in solving these problems. Roughly 15 million Americans suffer from some kind of food allergy, and that statistic includes 1 in 13 kids. In fact, between 1997 and 2011, childhood food allergy rates rose by 50 percent in the United States alone. Something is going on here.

 YOU ARE WHAT YOU EAT

GMOs are very controversial these days, and with good reason. We're not talking about the kind of genetic conditioning that's been done for centuries, like creating hybrid plants within a species or coercing animals with desirable traits to breed. We're talking about the deliberate insertion of foreign DNA into a plant. The Human Genome Project has discovered that the way genes work is vastly more complex than previously thought. Claiming that it's safe and predictable to insert DNA from bacteria and viruses into plants is simply untrue. We don't know what kind of rogue proteins could eventually be produced in these processes. That's why choosing non-GMO products is a wise choice for your gut health.

What has changed so much in the production of food in the past couple of decades that might explain such drastic increases in allergies? One theory is related to the widespread use of an herbicide called glyphosate that became one of the bestselling chemicals used in commercial farming in the early 1980s. It's now used extensively worldwide on sugar, corn, wheat, and soy and leaves a residue on all of these foods. A recent study in Europe found levels of the herbicide in people from 18 different countries. These alarming discoveries helped precipitate bans on the substance in several European countries, and others are following suit. So if glyphosate contamination is both widespread and controversial, why is it still be used? Glyphosate is considered harmless to humans, so it continues to get a safety pass in most countries. But guess who is highly sensitive to its damaging effects? You guessed it, our gut microbes.

The worst thing about glyphosate is the decimating effect it has on the beneficial bacteria in our gut. The chemical actually prefers to attack the good microbes in our gut and practically guarantees the pathogens will run amok. There is no doubt that glyphosate contributes to the rise of inflammatory and allergic conditions. Your microbiome cells outnumber your own by 10 to 1, and every single one of those microbes is susceptible to the damaging effects of this widely used herbicide. Without a healthy microbe population, the immune system is crippled. Let's look at how this happens.

Your Peyer's patches—those nodules of lymphatic tissue on the intestinal wall—are like the guards at the castle gates. They see pathogens and take them into custody (literally by absorbing them). Then the pathogens get passed along to white blood cells and presented to specialized T-cells that decide if what they're dealing with is a friend or foe. The T-cells then alert the rest of your immune cells to launch a body-wide response. When toxins like glyphosate run rampant through your system, there are too many pathogens in which to respond. Add the increased intestinal permeability and potential tight-junction malfunction induced by the imbalance, and you have a recipe for allergies and inflammation.

The same Th1 and Th2 immune cell issues we discussed earlier that lead to autoimmunity can also stimulate Immunoglobulin E (IgE) production. IgE is the antibody in charge of allergic reactions. Once your altered microbiome negatively affects your T-cells, you might be producing too much IgE. Immunoglobulin E binds to allergens and signals the *mast cells* in the *connective tissues* of your body to release substances that cause inflammation. When IgE also binds to the mast cells themselves, you get full-blown allergic reactions like hives, runny nose, sneezing, and itchiness.

> **DEFINITION**
>
> Cells in the connective tissues of your body that release substances in response to inflammation or injury are called **mast cells. Connective tissues** bind, support, or separate tissues and organs, and are made up of proteins such as collagen.

Everyone's bodies are wired differently according to their own unique environmental exposures to different toxins (like glyphosate) and antigens coupled with their genetics. Research has revealed clostridia bacteria in particular play a role in protecting us against allergic responses by sending messages to immune cells to produce molecules that reduce intestinal permeability. Once the gut microbiome is out of balance however, these bacteria can't perform those functions. When immune system function and the intestinal wall are compromised, IgE is free to react against antigens in the blood unchecked. Allergies can range from annoying to life-threatening, but they're set into motion by compromised gut health.

Respiratory Diseases

There is some overlap in the causes of allergies, inflammatory responses, and respiratory disease. One of the substances IgE can trigger your mast cells to release is a neurotransmitter called histamine. Histamine can induce inflammatory, allergic, and respiratory responses. (You might have even taken an "antihistamine" to prevent your own body from releasing histamine during allergy season.) The neurotransmitter causes smooth muscles to contract and blood vessels to swell. This is supposed to help white blood cells find the source of an injury, but it can give you a headache, cause itchiness, fatigue, difficulty breathing (think allergy season again), and generally make you miserable.

GUT WISE

Studies suggest that a diverse population of microbes in the guts of infants helps protect them from developing asthma. The lower the diversity in the gut, the higher the asthma risk. The microbes in a developing infant actually instruct the baby's immune cells. Without all the members of the gut microbe drill sergeant team, the immunity army doesn't get trained as well and overreacts to harmless substances.

There are a number of cells that naturally produce histamines, but there are also pathogenic bacteria that produce them as well. Certain strains of E. coli and staphylococci are some of the most famous culprits. If these bacteria overgrow, the histamine they produce seeps into the circulatory system and causes a wide range of symptoms, one of which is respiratory difficulties. Histamine can cause muscles in your airways to contract and make your *bronchioles* too narrow. Inflammation in the lung tissue, histamine, or other sources, compound the breathing problem. These are the underlying causes of asthma attacks and other respiratory conditions.

Eating Disorders

We include a discussion of eating disorders, such as bulimia and anorexia, to build another bridge between the topics of physical and mental health. Although eating disorders are largely treated with psychological counseling and care, the gut microbiota can also play a role. Like we've said before, those little organisms affect nearly every aspect of health.

DEFINITION

Your lungs have main airways that branch off into smaller airways called **bronchioles** that end in tiny air sacs called alveoli. **Anorexia nervosa** is an eating disorder characterized by the patient's refusal of food, a distorted body image or **body dysmorphia,** and an obsession with losing weight. **Bulimia** has all of the symptoms of anorexia, but in addition is coupled with periods of binge eating, self-induced vomiting, and fasting.

When someone suffers an eating disorder, they inevitably develop nutrient deficiencies. These deficiencies lead to immune system problems that leave the body vulnerable to infections. Often these infections need to be treated with antibiotics, which further disrupt gut bacteria populations. The toxic build-up of pathogenic bacteria and their by-products exacerbate and/or lead to leaky gut and leaky blood-brain barrier. Your blood-brain barrier does for your brain and spinal cord what your intestinal lining does for the gut. The blood-brain barrier is a system of capillaries that act like a filter, keeping the bad stuff out. But if this barrier is leaky, then toxins can breach the filter.

Some theories suggest that *body dysmorphia* might be the result of toxins from pathogenic bacteria and their by-products altering sensory perception in the brain. Body dysmorphia is a condition that causes patients to see themselves as fat when they're really thin.

The gut dysbiosis in an anorexic or bulimic irritates the gut lining and interrupts the cycle of enterocyte regeneration. This hinders the patient's ability to digest food and absorb nutrients. When the anorexic or bulimic then tries to eat a little something, they suffer all kinds of digestive distress. People suffering from eating disorders should work to heal their gut alongside the psychological treatments they receive for their conditions. A healed and sealed gut lining will stop the flow of toxins, which may contribute to their body dysmorphia. Psychotherapy will do wonders in helping them heal emotionally, and probiotics, bone broths (see Chapter 11), and other proper nourishment will help them soothe and restore their gut lining as they achieve healthier attitudes toward food.

 YOU ARE WHAT YOU EAT

> Not only does eating refined sugars feed unhealthy gut bacteria, it also leads to inflammation in the body, including the brain. Taking in all the probiotics and bone broth in the world will not make a difference if you do not cut back on the refined sugars.

Mental Health

The brain-gut axis provides a constant flow of signals and substances traveling a two-way street. Our gut microbiota produce neurotransmitters and other substances that travel along the vagus nerve. If something is amiss at either end of the "highway," the other end will know about it. Our microbes produce by-products that cross the blood-brain barrier. Our brain sends signals to the "second brain," which is the enteric nervous system of our gut. Again, the interconnectivity is becoming clearer.

Although the *exact* mechanisms of how microbiota manifest specific neurological and/or psychological conditions haven't been discovered yet, the scientific foundation is there. The connection is real. Our gut is our second brain and has the capacity to affect our mood, cognitive function, and our behavior. Unraveling the intricacies of these connections will help us gain a better understanding and command of our mental health.

Gut-Brain Axis and Emotional Health

When you were a fetus, a clump of tissue called the neural crest divided into two parts. One part became the central nervous system, and the other became the enteric nervous system of your gut. They're like twins separated at birth that still talk to each other via a "phone" line called the vagus nerve. Ever hear those crazy stories involving separated twins when one is injured and the other feels the pain even though they're miles apart? You have something just as fascinating going on inside of you right now.

Many studies have illustrated the gut-brain connection. Even your positive outlook on life or negativity has this two-way influence. A healthy well-balanced gut is routinely associated with a sunny disposition, and depression and mental illness have been linked to low-diversity gut microbiomes and gut dysbiosis.

GUT WISE

While you sleep, your brain waves move in cycles of 90 minutes worth of slow waves interrupted by rapid eye movement or REM sleep, which is when dreams occur. Your "second brain" in the gut generates 90 minute cycles of slow contractions interrupted by short, quick muscle contractions. Interestingly, people with abnormal gut issues also have abnormal REM cycles. Perhaps Grandma was right when she said not to have a snack right before bed. It might give you nightmares after all.

In 2001, *The Journal of Clinical Psychiatry* released a survey that concluded 50 to 90 percent of IBS patients also suffered from a psychiatric condition such as anxiety disorders, depression, and post-traumatic stress disorder (PTSD). Emotional trauma in general can cause gut-brain axis sensitivities. People with IBD (including Crohn's disease) also have lesions on the brain with similar frequency as those with multiple sclerosis. All of these conditions are related because they all involve inflammation, immune dysfunction, intestinal hyperpermeability, and of course, the microbe connection to all of those factors.

Gut microbiota cause neurochemical changes in the brain, which in turn can influence behavior. Behavioral development is most certainly influenced by the health and diversity of gut microbiota. One of your body's main regulators of mood and social behaviors is serotonin, a neurotransmitter that helps nerve cells communicate with one another. Your gut makes 95 percent of the serotonin in your body. And guess what helps? Your mighty microbes. So quite literally, if your gut isn't happy and behaving nicely, neither are you.

> **YOU ARE WHAT YOU EAT**
>
> Amino acids are crucial to helping you produce enough serotonin to improve your emotional well-being. Eating more glycine-rich foods can help balance out the amino acid ratios needed to make sure the building blocks for serotonin are readily absorbed by the body. The skin, cartilage, and bones of animals are perfect sources of glycine. Traditional bone broths provide lots of these nourishing substances. (See recipes for bone broths in Chapter 14.) You can also take gelatin supplements as well.

Numerous scientific studies over the past 30 years have demonstrated how gut microbes influence behavior and induce chemical changes in the brain. Pathogenic bacteria can obviously cause problems in this department, and experiments suggest that too many bad microbes in the gut can cause symptoms of anxiety. If you add immune dysfunction and inflammation to this pathogenic soup, you set the stage for chronic depression. Inflammation in the gut lining causes your gut to secrete cytokines, which communicate to white blood cells that it's time to produce inflammation. These cytokines can cross the blood-brain barrier and induce depression in sensitive individuals.

The good news about mood disorders and the gut is that if microbiota imbalance, inflammation, and leaky gut impact our mental health, then we most likely have much more control over mental illness than previously thought. The nervous system is a lot more flexible than science used to recognize. The brain-gut axis can be coaxed out of its bad habits if we heal it with proper nutrition protocols.

Microbiota and Extreme Mental Illness

The majority of patients who suffer from severe mental illnesses like schizophrenia, also have a history of digestive issues. New scientific studies have emerged over the past decade that show a link between gut dysbiosis (imbalance where there are more pathogenic bacteria than good) and psychiatric disorders. What's ironic about these "new" discoveries is that the older psychiatric literature, and even textbooks on the subject from the 1930s, routinely mentions connections between gut health and mental illness, specifically malnutrition. As it turns out, schizophrenic patients in particular are often suffer numerous vitamin and mineral deficiencies related to their gut microbiota imbalances.

An imbalance in the gut can lead to untold amounts of neurotoxins that are the by-product of bacteria's metabolism. Those toxins can seep into the bloodstream via a damaged and hyper-permeable intestinal lining. When these toxins get to the brain, they can wreak havoc. One of these toxins is the infamous candida. If this yeast population gets out of control, it interrupts the normal digestion of sugars and carbs in the body. It steals the sugars and instead of letting the body convert them into the lactic acid and energy it needs, it ferments the sugars instead. This dysfunctional process actually produces ethanol and acetaldehyde.

Ethanol is alcohol. Candida toxicity can leave a person with all the symptoms of drunkenness, and even alcoholism, without ever having guzzled an alcoholic beverage. In addition to the physical effects of persistent alcohol levels in the body, the mental effects are equally devastating including brain damage, lack of self-control, poor speech and coordination, altered senses, and interactions with medications.

Remember what we said in Chapter 6 about the consumption of milk and gluten in people with unhealthy microbiota? The microvilli of a healthy small intestine will break down the milk and gluten proteins into amino acids. So in people with mental illness, and therefore gut dysbiosis by default, these proteins get launched into the circulatory system.

In a broad spectrum of mental and cognitive disorders, the digestive systems convert milk protein (casein) and gluten into opiate-like substances called gluteomorphins and casomorphins. These natural opiates can disrupt normal brain function and development and negatively impact the immune system. Gluteomorphins and casomorphins have been detected in clinical urinalyses of patients with depression, Down's syndrome, severe postpartum depression, schizophrenia, attention deficit hyperactivity disorder (ADHD), and even some autoimmune disorders like rheumatoid arthritis (RA).

American Physician Dr. Curtis Dohan published a paper in 1988, titled "Genetic Hypothesis of Idiopathic Schizophrenia: Its Exorphin Connection." In his research, Dr. Dohan renewed interest in the connection between gluten, casein (milk protein), and the opiate-like substances they produce, and leaky gut and schizophrenia. He also studied cultures in the South Pacific, where people had never eaten gluten. Zero cases of schizophrenia were noted there. His recommendation? Remove gluten and casein from the diets of at-risk patients as early as possible to improve their chances of recovery.

It's really not a huge stretch to consider the implications of gut population on our mental health. Their cells outnumber ours 10 to 1. Their genes outnumber our own by 100 to 1. In a way, you could say that we're more bacteria than we are human. The best news about all of these connections is that even severe psychiatric conditions, and even cognitive disorders, can at least be mitigated from trying to heal the gut.

GUT WISE

Arachidonic acid (AA) is an omega-6 essential fatty acid that makes up about 12 percent of all fat in the brain. People with autism, depression, schizophrenia, and bipolar disorder have low AA levels. This interferes with the entire body because it disrupts all the processes and communications along the brain-gut axis. AA is found naturally in meat, eggs, and dairy products. Processed sugars and carbohydrates leech fatty acids from cell membranes, so it's important to avoid those foods and make sure you get a healthy combination of fatty acids from nuts, seeds (like pumpkin and chia), and fish oils.

Learning Disorders and Brain Function

Twenty years ago, autism affected 1 in 10,000 children, now it's 1 in 150 in both the United Kingdom and United States. When you evaluate the gut microbial composition of an autistic child, you will undoubtedly find dysbiosis. This is bad news for autism and other cognitive disorders, because studies show a direct correlation between diverse gut bacteria and higher learning scores. In order to lessen the effects of any learning disability or cognitive disorder, the gut bacteria balance has to be addressed.

Strains of clostridia most likely play a role in autism. In 1998, a case study at Great Plains Laboratories in Kansas revealed that administering courses of anticlostridia drugs made children with autism asymptomatic and improved their digestion. Unfortunately, the drugs have toxic side effects and could not be given over the long term. As soon as patients stopped taking the drug their symptoms would return.

Another gut balance issue in the autistic population is the overgrowth of sulfate-reducing bacteria. The body needs sulfates for processes that help with detoxification and brain neurotransmitters. Too many sulfate-reducing bacteria effectively steal sulfur from the gut and convert it into toxic substances. But the good news here is that gut microbiome rebalancing is a critical and viable option in treating autism.

There is little doubt that gut microbiota imbalance is at the root of the brain-gut axis problems plaguing those with autism and learning disabilities. The cycle is particularly hard to break because the abnormal gut microbes actually cause the afflicted person to crave sweet and starchy products that will further feed the pathogenic bacteria. These cravings are so strong that people with autism and learning disabilities will often refuse any other types of food.

There's a lot of evidence that these craving-inducing pathogens can breach the blood-brain barrier. The ensuing "brain fog" actually disrupts nerve signals about taste and texture causing even further pickiness. Making matters worse is that these same bacteria, especially candida, can alter taste bud function because toxins released by these bacteria get stored in the mouth's mucous membranes. This toxic dumping causes some nutrient-rich foods such as raw vegetables, fruit, nuts, and seeds to irritate the person's mouth. The end result is another food aversion and more pickiness.

These same cycles can also induce attention deficit disorder (ADD), attention deficit hyperactivity disorder (ADHD), and a general lack of focus. This is obviously disastrous for school-age children trying to perform academically. Compounding the problem of brain fog is the manic blood-sugar roller coaster that many of our children try to navigate unsuccessfully. The gut can quickly digest and absorb processed carbs, which are among kids' favorite foods, and the pathogenic bacteria are quick to help. Children's bodies then pump out insulin to handle the spike in blood sugar, and an hour later they crave even more simple carbs and sugar.

This sugar mania can produce highs and lows that cause some children to act out; hyperactivity and behavioral problems ensue.

GUT WISE

More than 90 percent of school-aged children in the United States don't eat the recommended daily servings of vegetables, and more than 75 percent don't eat enough fruit. But over 90 percent consume more than the recommended limits of fats and sugars. What children eat can directly correspondence to how they perform in school. In 2009, the University of Alberta in Canada studied the nutritional habits of 5,000 children. Kids who ate the recommended amounts of vegetables, fruit, protein, and dietary fiber tested better than their counterparts who ate less healthful foods—high in salt and fats.

Children with compromised intestinal linings and abnormal gut microbes often have pathogens roaming their entire bodies taking a toll on multiple systems, including the nervous system and brain. They may not develop the number of synaptic connections in their brains as other kids whose brain-gut axes are intact. The brain of a leaky gut child can misfire when he or she tries to master the tasks of reading and writing. It's not uncommon for children with ADD, ADHD, and dyslexia to also have typical leaky gut symptoms that parents may not realize are all connected.

Early childhood development is crucial to future academic success, and it's not unusual for children with leaky guts to fall behind in school. The toxic load they carry in their bodies often leads to processing disorders and learning disabilities. The way their brain gathers and processes sensory input is often disrupted, making classroom settings difficult on multiple levels.

These children need a multifaceted approach at home and at school, which involves behavior modification and a dietary regimen that reestablishes healthy gut microbes. They need to follow nutrition protocols to heal and seal the gut lining. A broad-based approach from parents and educators can help these children rewire their behavioral patterns while they literally learn to feed themselves the right kinds of foods. Once the beneficial bacteria get a chance to flourish, picky eating habits dissipate, brain fog clears, healthy communication along the vagus nerve is established, and real progress can be made.

The Least You Need to Know

- The state of your digestive health affects every other system in your body.
- Your gut microbiota work in conjunction with your immune system. If they're not diverse and in a state of homeostasis, autoimmune disorders may result.
- Gut dysbiosis can cause inflammation throughout the body, including the skin.
- The brain-gut axis is an undeniable study in interconnectivity; what affects one affects the other.
- Gut microbes help produce the serotonin that plays a role in your mood and behavior.
- Establishing a diverse and well-balanced population of gut microbiota is crucial in treating mental illness and cognitive disorders.

CHAPTER 8

Gut Aggravators

In this chapter, we take a closer look at aggravators of the gut. The drugs we take routinely for disease maintenance and to fight infections may alleviate symptoms in the short term, but what are the effects on our digestive system? We'll also examine some self-medicating drugs of choice like alcohol and caffeine, parasitic gut invaders, and a major enemy we all need to conquer—stress!

In This Chapter

- Common medications that damage gut lining and microbiota
- Ways alcohol consumption affects gut health
- The dangers of intestinal parasites
- How stress takes a toll on your gut

Medications

Modern life has its advantages, and creature comforts are high on most people's wish list. Science and medicine have joined forces in the developing world to help us keep pain and suffering at bay, or at least to better manage it. Even minor discomforts that were simply endured for centuries are now mitigated by the proliferation of over-the-counter drugs. Got a headache? Pop this pill. Heartburn? Down a cup of this liquid. Tired? Take this to keep you awake.

For more serious diseases, the list of pharmaceutical cocktails is more extensive, and not without considerable risks that must be weighed again the benefits. A favorite cultural meme is the laundry list of side effects read off at 100 miles per hour near the end of every drug commercial aired on network television. Have you noticed how many gastrointestinal side effects get rattled off? Constipation, diarrhea, abdominal pain, intestinal cramping, anal leakage. It's quite a list.

One of the first things they teach doctors in pharmacology classes in medical school is that all drugs are toxic. We just decide the dose we're willing to tolerate and what side effects are acceptable. Any drug in our body is a foreign substance. Sometimes they have lifesaving properties for which we're grateful. Sometimes they aren't necessary and shouldn't really be our go-to solution for problems that could be remedied with food, exercise, and rest.

> **GUT WISE**
>
> Medical students at universities in both Europe and the United States spend anywhere between 4 to 60 times the number of hours on studying the effects of drugs in the body than they do studying nutrition.

Our desire for immediate gratification in every aspect of our lives clouds our judgment in both personal and professional health care. There are often long-term consequences for these conveniences and freedom from temporary discomfort. One of the main consequences is compromised gut health.

Painkillers

One of the most commonly used pain relief and fever-reducing medications in the world is acetaminophen ("paracetamol" in Europe). You probably know it by the brand name Tylenol and by its reputation as one of the safest medications you can take. It's one of the few over-the-counter (OTC) drugs rated as safe for pregnant women and infants.

This medicine, however, has risks and can cause liver damage if taken incorrectly. Even if taken regularly, it can also be a gut aggravator. Doses of 2,000 milligrams a day or more put you at an increased risk of bleeding or perforation in your esophagus, stomach, and small intestine (your upper GI tract). There are also cases of nausea and vomiting with the higher doses people take regularly to manage chronic pain. Another reason to limit this drug is that scientists are still debating how it works in our bodies. They understand the results and the effects of its toxicity in high doses, but they're not exactly sure *how* it blocks our pain.

Drugs in the opiate family are actually better understood. Medicines classified as opiates include morphine, tramadol, methadone, codeine, and oxycodone. These are much stronger painkillers that are usually prescribed after trauma or surgery. Even in the short term, these drugs can take a toll on the GI tract. They can cause nausea, dry mouth, bloating, acid reflux, immune system problems, and constipation. The constipation can be severe and painful, often lasting for the duration the drug is prescribed. It's very common for people on prescription opiates to also be advised to take laxatives.

Long-term opiate use has been known to damage nerves in the gut so that any abdominal pain is intensified. People who abuse opioids can end up with what some doctors call narcotic bowel syndrome (NBS). This can lead to serious stomach cramping and make withdrawal from the drugs especially difficult.

The bottom line on this class of drugs is that they really should only be used in the smallest effective doses to ease the pain associated with trauma and postsurgical recovery. This is especially important given their addictive nature. Staying on these types of medications long term damages your gut's ability to perform peristalsis (muscle contractions) normally, to effectively monitor intestinal transit time, to produce comfortable bowel movements, and to conduct normal communication with the brain.

Corticosteroids and NSAIDs

Corticosteroids and nonsteroidal anti-inflammatory drugs (NSAIDs) are both used to combat inflammation in the body. Their side effects include the impairment of kidney function, interfering with proper blood clotting, digestive system discomfort, and GI tract injury. Both of these drug classes are aggravators of the gut.

Corticosteroids fight inflammation in the body by suppressing the immune system. Common medicines in this group are prednisone, methylprednisolone, and cortisone. One of the ways corticosteroids reduce your immune system's inflammatory responses is by interrupting cytokine production. Without the cytokines secreting from white blood cells to stimulate the rally cry to other white cells to congregate at the site of a perceived injury or infection, the inflammation in the body is reduced.

Corticosteroids also diminish your body's ability to make antibodies; this hinders the activity of IgE and other immunoglobulins that act out against food particles or healthy tissues. They also suppress the specialized white blood cells called macrophages that have the ability to travel to the site of infection and engulf and destroy pathogens. Corticosteroids also slow the production of other pro-inflammatory substances in the body. The problem here is that the real cause of the inflammation hasn't been taken away, only the body's response to it has. The other issue is that if a legitimate invader gets into your body, your immune system can't respond normally. You are more vulnerable to contagious infections when you take these steroids, and this includes intestinal and GI infections, in general.

Corticosteroids take a toll on your digestive system in both the short and long term. They often irritate the gut mucosa. They raise blood sugar and disrupt metabolism by making you feel hungrier than normal and retain water.

Corticosteroids also damage the gut microbiota. They kill off some beneficial bacteria while feeding candida. You also double your risk of upper GI bleeding and perforation when you take steroids. If you take a steroid and an NSAID together, you are 12 times more likely to develop upper GI complications like bleeding.

Sometimes these medications are necessary to combat pain and inflammation in the body when they become unmanageable, and you need relief. Knowing the risks can help motivate you to work on the real sources of inflammation in your body so that you can safely wean yourself off the potentially harmful long-term use of these medications.

GUT WISE

Approximately 107,000 people are hospitalized for GI tract issues from NSAID use in the United States every year. In fact, 81 percent of them had no previous gastrointestinal symptoms or complaints before the sudden onset of internal bleeding that sent them rushing for emergency care. At least 16,500 rheumatoid and osteoarthritis patients die from prescription NSAID GI complications annually in the United States.

Nonsteroidal anti-inflammatory drugs are exactly what they sound like—substances that are not steroids but are used to combat inflammation in the body. Common OTC drugs in this category are aspirin, naproxen, and ibuprofen (known by the brand names Bayer, Aleve, and Advil, respectively). People take these drugs regularly for minor pain and fever relief. Daily doses of prescription NSAIDs, such as Celebrex, are often recommended for people suffering with moderate to severe arthritis and other chronic pain conditions.

Every year in the United States alone, more than 70 million prescriptions are written for NSAIDs. Additionally, Americans buy over 30 billion OTC doses of these drugs annually. There's obviously an enormous demand for anti-inflammatory relief, and because so many of these drugs are being ingested, it's important to be educated about their effects on our bodies.

NSAIDs cause widespread bodily damage because they harm cell membranes and interrupt crucial functions inside cells such as energy production. They also specifically target the lining of the gut. Clinical research has demonstrated that NSAID usage actually increases intestinal permeability, contributing to leaky gut. Additionally, if you take NSAIDs, you're four times more likely to develop internal bleeding in your upper GI tract. The risk is even more than that when you combine different anti-inflammatory drugs, especially corticosteroids. Approximately 60 percent of people who take NSAIDs regularly for arthritis alone will have some kind of adverse side effect from the drugs. Stomach ulcers are among the most common of these negative consequences.

So how do NSAIDs do this kind of damage? They inhibit the production of mucous and a bicarbonate-rich substance that protects our stomach lining from its own acid, and they interrupt blood circulation necessary for cell repair and renewal in the stomach lining. NSAIDs block these processes by blocking the production of an ulcer-preventing enzyme called *cyclooxygenase-1* (COX-1). This enzyme contributes to the production of *prostaglandins,* which are fatty acids that act like hormones in our body. These substances play a role in muscle contraction, blood vessel movement, blood-pressure regulation, and inflammation control. Prostaglandins are also produced in response to cell injury. NSAIDs stop that production, and in that way can have a negative impact on your immune system in general.

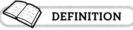 **DEFINITION**

> **Prostaglandins** are substances in your body which act like hormones and help modulate inflammation in the body. **Cyclooxygenase-1 (COX-1)** is an enzyme used by the body to make prostaglandins and is essential for stomach and kidney health.

Low prostaglandin and COX-1 production have specific impacts on your digestive health. When you take NSAIDs, the COX-1 that would normally help increase blood circulation to the stomach needed for mucous and cell repair just doesn't happen. The stomach lining is then wide open for acid erosion, irritation, and the development of ulcers. If you just take an Aleve or Advil every once in a while, the stomach will heal itself and you won't suffer long-term side effects. It's the people who use these drugs regularly for chronic symptoms or the slightest discomfort that will bear the brunt of negative GI side effects. Ulcers that can't heal because the COX-1 continues to be inhibited by NSAIDs can bleed. This can quickly turn into a life-threatening condition.

If you're taking NSAIDs and you notice any of these symptoms, stop taking them and seek medical attention:

- Stomach pain that feels like a burning in the abdomen—it may come on suddenly and then disappear for hours at a time before recurring

- Loss of appetite

- Persistent nausea

- Stomach pain that temporarily goes away upon eating, only to return an hour or so later

- Black or tarry stools (This usually indicates internal bleeding.)

- Fatigue (This could indicate bleeding ulcers.)

- Vomiting blood (This is a sure sign your ulcers are bleeding and require immediate emergency medical treatment.)

As with corticosteroids and painkillers, it's important to know the risks, especially to your digestive system. Working to find the source of inflammation is always better than simply masking the symptoms with drugs whose side effects may often be worse in the long run than the symptoms you wanted to lessen in the first place.

Antacids, Acid-Reducers, and Proton Pump Inhibitors

Most of us have reached for an OTC indigestion medication at one time or another, especially in a culture that overindulges on a number of special occasions. The ads for these products are often humorous depictions of uncomfortable people who have stuffed themselves and suffer the bloated consequences. We often look at these images and laugh because we've been there. The problem with drugs that control stomach acid however, lies in their regular use.

There are three major kinds of stomach acid control medications: antacids, H2 blockers (acid-reducers), and proton pump inhibitors (PPIs). Antacids typically contain calcium carbonate or a combination of aluminum hydroxide and magnesium carbonate. These medicines neutralize the acid in your stomach quickly. H2 blockers reduce the amount of acid your stomach produces and work for longer periods of time than antacids. These acid-blockers usually contain ranitidine or famotidine. Proton pump inhibitors drastically reduce the amount of acid in your stomach and are generally recommended for people with chronic acid reflux. Common PPIs contain omeprazole or lansoprazole.

Between 2001 and 2010, prescriptions written for PPIs doubled. Proton pump inhibitors were so commonly prescribed for an equally common acid reflux condition, that they are now available over the counter. Their use is so pervasive we need to evaluate their impact on gut health. The ironic thing about the use of acid-reducers and neutralizers is that most people who take them have the opposite problem. The overproduction of acid in the stomach is a much rarer condition than we think. About half of us actually suffer from too *little* acid, a condition known as *hypochlorhydria*. Some of us take medications meant for high stomach acid because the symptoms of both high and low stomach acid are similar.

> **DEFINITION**
>
> If your stomach and other digestive organs do not produce enough of the gastric secretion called hydrochloric acid then you suffer from **hypochlorhydria.**

Bloating, reflux, constipation, and indigestion symptoms are typical if you have hypochlorhydria because food is sitting in the stomach undigested for too long. But beyond being uncomfortable, hypochlorhydria can result in vitamin and mineral deficiencies because some of these substances require a lot of stomach acid to be absorbed by our digestive system. Magnesium, iron, copper, calcium, zinc, folic acid, vitamin B_{12}, and proteins all need higher levels of stomach acid for proper absorption. Common heartburn medications inhibit protein digestion, which in turn hinders the absorption of these key nutrients.

Stomach acid also plays a vital role in our immune system. If we ingest a food-borne pathogen or parasite, the stomach acid kills them before we can get sick. The acid also kills any bacteria that make their way up from the small intestine to try to colonize the stomach. People with low stomach acid are therefore more vulnerable to food poisoning, candida overgrowth, and SIBO that spills over into the stomach.

Getting stomach acid levels balanced is critical for a healthy gut. This may leave you wondering, "If the symptoms for low acid and high acid are similar, how do I figure out which one I have?" This is an excellent question, and one in which you should invest some time, and some money, to get correctly answered. This means professional medical consultation. If you are one of the few people who actually have too much acid and you don't address it properly, you run the risk of serious problems like esophageal erosion that can lead to cancer. The good news is there is a conclusive medical test that can give you an answer about the exact composition of your stomach acid. The bad news is most insurance companies don't cover it.

The Heidelberg Stomach Acid Test costs around $350 without insurance. But it will give you results you can use to determine if you need to take medications to control acid production or if you need to take supplements to actually stimulate more stomach acid (such as Betaine HCL with pepsin). The test involves going off your acid-reducers or neutralizers for 4 days. Then you fast overnight (or for 8 to 12 hours) and swallow a pill with a transmitter inside that can read the exact pH of your stomach. You then drink a sodium bicarbonate solution (basically baking soda) and the transmitter will record your stomach acid production over whatever time period your health-care practitioner deems appropriate in your circumstance. This is the ultimate test for conclusive results about whether or not you have too much or too little stomach acid. Once you know the root of the problem, you can take the best steps toward a healthier gut.

Antidepressants

According to the National Center for Health Statistics, 1 in every 10 Americans has a prescription for an antidepressant. Between 1988 and 2008, the number of Americans over the age of 12 who take these medications increased by nearly 400 percent. They are some of the most commonly prescribed drugs and make more money than any other class of medication in the United States. Again, with drugs this pervasive, we must evaluate their side effects, especially as aggravators of the gut.

Many antidepressant medications increase serotonin levels. These are called selective serotonin reuptake inhibitors (SSRIs). Infants born to pregnant women taking SSRIs, as well as children prescribed SSRIs at an early age, are prone to further mood disorders later in life. This will put them at risk for further side effects from potentially more medications. SSRIs themselves cause negative GI side effects, the most common being nausea. SSRIs also cause abdominal cramping, diarrhea, acid reflux, constipation, dry mouth, and general indigestion. Some side effects of these medications cause long-term structural damage to the body and brain. Other side effects cause acute damage to the gut lining and are similar to the GI bleeding caused by many NSAIDs.

> **GUT WISE**
>
> Despite the vast differences in cost, antidepressants have been shown to be equally effective across the board. In other words, there really isn't one that's better than all the others. There have also been numerous clinical studies that show antidepressants aren't that much more effective than placebos in the majority of individuals tested. These findings offer more food for thought when weighing the health risks with the possible benefits of antidepressants.

One enormous problem of antidepressant side effects is that they're often managed with further prescription drugs. SSRIs (like Prozac) often cause feelings of anxiousness, so they're often administered alongside doses of sedatives to balance out the patient. These sedatives (like benzodiazapine) often cause marked drowsiness and can lead to even further depression. Because so many SSRIs cause GI irritation, including bleeding ulcers, doctors often prescribe acid-reducers to prevent that from happening. As we know, those drugs used over the long term have their own list of side effects. Again, caution must be exercised when dealing with these drugs.

Antibiotics

Antibiotics are the most commonly prescribed medications in the world. We are also exposed, although the science is conflicted as to the degree, through the antibiotics routinely given to the animals raised on commercial farms. There is no doubt that antibiotics are lifesaving substances in combatting virulent infections. But the pervasive use of these drugs for low-risk infections may be more damaging than toughing out lower-risk infections now and then.

So how do antibiotics aggravate the gut? They disrupt the natural balance of microbiota, as we have previously discussed. They can also cause general stomach upset and diarrhea. One the most serious problems that can arise from antibiotic use is the overgrowth of *Clostridium difficile,* and the diarrhea induced by that pathogen can be life-threatening. Penicillin (which includes amoxicillin, clindamycin, and cephalosporins) is the most likely antibiotic culprit to spark a *Clostridium difficile* overgrowth.

Antibiotics in general kill off beneficial bacteria, which causes an overgrowth of pathogenic strains. Some benign viruses and fungi in the microbiome even convert to pathogenic varieties when they come into contact with antibiotics and start invading healthy tissues. The irony of antibiotics is their damaging effects on the gut microbiota can compromise our immune system and make us vulnerable to infections that require more powerful antibiotics to fight.

Some of the most common antibiotics are derived from penicillin. These drugs kill off lactobacilli and bifidobacteria and promote pathogenic strains of strep and staph infections. Penicillin-based antibiotics allow bacteria that usually only live in the colon to travel up to the small intestine where they can cause a person to develop serious digestive problems and even diseases like IBS.

GUT WISE

Candida runs rampant in the gut nearly every time a broad-spectrum antibiotic enters the body. Doctors know this and used to routinely prescribe Nystatin every time a course of antibiotics was given. This antifungal drug would kill off candida while the antibiotic killed the infection. For reasons unknown, this practice is not as common, but talk with your doctor about your candida concerns, and he'll most likely write you that nystatin prescription alongside your antibiotic.

Tetracyclines are a family of antibiotics often prescribed for acne. These drugs are a real issue for the gut because they're usually taken over long periods, sometimes as long as 2 years. A lot of gut aggravation can happen in that time. Tetracycline leaves the gut wall vulnerable to attack from pathogenic bacteria because it alters the structure of mucous membranes, including the gut mucosa. The immune system then launches an attack against these changed proteins, which can trigger autoimmunity in the gut. In short, tetracycline can cause your gut wall to start attacking itself.

Caffeine

Caffeine is a stimulant. So many of us are addicted to the kick-start caffeine can give to our mornings (or the middle of the afternoon). The prospect of giving that up can be intimidating. But the reality is that caffeine operates much more like a drug than a food substance and is a known stomach agitator.

Remember the stomach acid issues we discussed earlier? Caffeine can trigger extra hydrochloric acid (HCL) production and cause too much acid, which can irritate the gut lining. Over time, however, caffeine ends up producing the opposite effect in "heavy users." The body's ability to keep churning out those high quantities of HCL diminishes with the overtaxing effects of caffeine. Then you're stuck with the nutrient absorption and bacteria disruption problems of hypochlorhydria. In fact, studies show that caffeine can inhibit the absorption of minerals such as magnesium and iron even in the short term.

As a stimulant, caffeine elevates the levels of adrenaline and cortisol in the blood. These stress hormones raise our blood pressure and quicken our pulse and basically make us feel jittery and anxious because they're part of our "fight or flight" response system. During those responses, our digestive system slows down considerably, and the end result is often indigestion from all the anxiety the hormones trigger.

As much as caffeine may slow down digestion, it still can produce laxative and diuretic effects and make you have to use the bathroom more frequently. These effects can be so pronounced in some people that it leads to dehydration and mineral loss. Additionally, caffeine relaxes the lower esophageal sphincter (LES) and causes acid reflux.

 YOU ARE WHAT YOU EAT

Caffeine drinkers tend to eat more often because they mistakenly read symptoms of their withdrawal as hunger pangs. Coffee, in particular, has some antioxidant properties and contains polyphenols, which are micronutrients known to aid in the prevention of cardiovascular disease and cancer. While there is this benefit, the key with coffee is a small dose. A cup of coffee a day is acceptable, while too much can be detrimental.

There is an upside to coffee consumption specifically. Studies show it actually increases the population of the beneficial gut microbe bifidobacterium. You'll have to decide for yourself if it's worth all the other literal aggravation to yield the same results you could get from ingesting healthier alternatives such as yogurt.

Alcohol

Humans most likely developed the capacity for breaking down alcohol millions of years ago so we could make the most of fermenting fruit that had fallen off trees on the ancient forest floors of our ancestors. Consuming small amounts of alcohol can actually have some beneficial effects, such as a decreased likelihood of gallstones, stroke, and heart disease. Moderation, however, is key.

GUT WISE

Although it's best for gut health to avoid alcohol altogether, it's hard to go through every holiday and celebration in life without at least some small indulgences. The spirits that are kindest to the gut are gin, scotch, whiskey, bourbon, and vodka. Dry wines are also okay in small doses. It puts the "special" in "special occasion." We all have to live a little; just think before you drink.

Everyone knows that too much alcohol is bad for the body. But for some people, it becomes a frequent indulgence for social or habitual reasons. Alcohol consumption overloads our livers with more toxins to filter and over time can lead to *cirrhosis*. It also takes a toll on the entire digestive system. Additionally, alcohol compounds the battle for gut homeostasis by encouraging the wrong kind of bacteria growth.

How Excessive Alcohol Consumption Affects the Digestive System

Alcohol in excess, as a result of alcoholism, causes damage along the entire GI tract. It increases the chances of getting mouth cancer and gum disease. Esophageal lining erosion can be caused by the acid reflux that alcoholism can induce. The lining of the stomach suffers consequences as well, as alcohol abuse can trigger *gastritis*, or inflammation of the stomach wall.

The small intestine isn't spared. High rates of alcohol consumption increase the risk of intestinal cancer and the damage to the gut wall can lead to or exacerbate a leaky gut and IBS symptoms, such as diarrhea and constipation. Alcohol further compromises the intestinal wall by damaging its ability to absorb nutrients. This is usually made worse because an alcoholic will feel full from drinking and lose interest in food due to a suppressed appetite. The malnutrition that results can be so severe that it leads to *peripheral neuropathy* and alcoholic dementia.

> **DEFINITION**
>
> **Cirrhosis** is caused by alcohol abuse or hepatitis. The disease affects the liver and is characterized by inflammation, cell damage and degeneration, and a thickening of organ tissue. Erosion, irritation, or inflammation of the stomach lining is known commonly as **gastritis. Peripheral neuropathy** happens as a result of nerve damage. It manifests as weakness, pain, and/or numbness primarily in the hands and feet, but it can occur elsewhere in the body. The pain is usually described as burning or stabbing.

How Alcohol Abuse Disrupts Gut Symbiosis

Chronic alcohol abuse can alter the population of gut microbes in your small intestine. Specifically it can lower your *Bacteroidetes*, which are the beneficial class of bacteria that play a role in healthy metabolism and the strains that contribute to the integrity of the intestinal wall by decreasing your chances of hyperpermeability. In this way, alcohol can contribute to a leaky gut and lead to autoimmune diseases.

In addition to killing off the good guys in the *Bacteroidetes* family, alcohol abuse promotes the growth of *Proteobacteria*. *Proteobacteria* are supposed to be kept in check by the normal population control mechanisms of gut homeostasis, but alcohol disrupts all of that. Pathogens in this family of bacteria include the harmful strains of E. coli and salmonella. The unchecked growth of these and other pathogens caused by alcohol-induced dysbiosis compromise both the intestinal wall and the blood-brain barrier. It isn't uncommon for alcoholics to also suffer from depression and neurological disorders.

Intestinal Parasites

Sometimes, through no fault of our own, invaders from outside our body hitchhike a ride into our gut on the food we eat. As gross as it may seem, this happens very commonly in the developed world as well as more remote places. Most people, regardless of where they live, are inhabited by some kind of intestinal parasite.

Unfortunately, these microscopic beings offer no health benefits like the best members of our microbiome do. A healthy immune system and intact intestinal wall will keep these bugs in their place, and they won't do much damage. But if we already suffer from a leaky gut, these little creatures can injure our digestive system.

Parasites fall into two categories: worms and protozoa. Tapeworms and roundworms are a group of parasites that attack our bodies by latching on to our gut lining and robbing us of nutrients. Moreover, their latching can lead to internal bleeding and anemia. People contract them by drinking contaminated water, eating undercooked meat, and in some cases absorbing them through the skin. Protozoa are one-celled organisms that usually induce diarrhea and stomach upset.

One of the most prevalent of protozoa is a creature called Giardia. Around 30 percent of workers and children in day-care facilities carry this parasite. Oftentimes, people are misdiagnosed with IBS when what they really suffer from is this protozoan infection. Giardia is astoundingly easy to get but easy to mistake for other GI conditions. Instances of Giardia contamination of water supplies have been documented, and the results were localized epidemics of diarrhea followed by subsequent epidemics of digestion and malnutrition problems that lead to conditions such as chronic fatigue syndrome. These issues persisted for months after the initial infection.

Protozoa and other parasites can usually coexist with us as long as their numbers aren't too high and our intestinal lining isn't hyperpermeable. Unfortunately if we already have a leaky gut, or if their numbers are high enough to cause damage to our intestinal wall, then illness is inevitable. A rampant parasite infection can actually induce leaky gut syndrome and usher in a wave of unprecedented allergies, inflammation, and autoimmunity.

Stress

We're told so often about the negative impact stress has on every aspect of our lives, but we often feel we're too busy to do something about it. And that feeling is a major part of the problem. So many studies show that if we take time out to decompress, exercise, and just spend a few minutes walking in the outdoors, we'd not only be less stressed, but we'd be even more productive. This idea still strikes us as counterintuitive in a world where we're often expected to answer work emails at 10 o'clock at night.

> **GUT WISE**
>
> Do you wake up in the middle of the night, but you can't fall back to sleep? Do you get lightheaded upon standing and need caffeine to keep you awake? Do you feel tired all day long? Do you crave carbs and possibly eat more than 50 percent of your calories after 5 P.M.? Do you suffer from depression, anxiety, nervousness, irritability, weight gain, sugar cravings, high blood pressure, and/or abnormal blood lipids? Do you have difficulty recovering from exercise? If so, you are likely suffering from high cortisol levels, a hormone released during periods of stress. Chronic elevated cortisol levels cause inflammation, thyroid, and metabolic disorders.

Gut Microbes and the Nervous System

There is more nervous tissue running its way through your gut than in your spinal column or your *peripheral nervous system*. Your gut mucosa contains blood vessels influenced by your autonomic nervous system and a whole network of nerves (called the myenteric plexus), which are embedded in the intestinal lining and are influenced by the brain. The modern scientific consensus seems to be that the complicated and far-reaching network of your enteric nervous system (ENS) evolved to do more than just ensure the work of digestion could be done independent of your brain.

> **DEFINITION**
>
> The **peripheral nervous system** is the network of nerves throughout the body that are outside your spinal column and brain and connect the rest of your body to the central nervous system.

The trillions of microbes living in your gut interact with your ENS. Together they play an active part in digestion as they both are involved with digestive enzyme production. The ENS sends the signals which control peristalsis that keeps material moving along your GI tract. The gut microbes also "communicate" with the brain via neurotransmitters and other substances that send signals back and forth between the gut and brain via the vagus nerve.

How Stress Affects the Gut (and Vice Versa)

Because of the extensive interconnectivity between your gut and brain, stress is going to take its toll on both. Even short periods of stress can upset the balance of your gut microbiota. The good news is that when the stressful event is over, your gut recovers. Maybe you've noticed this yourself when you're stressed out about something. Your stomach feels like it's in knots, but once you find closure or resolution, then you feel more relaxed and so does your gut.

Stress can induce and exacerbate digestive problems. It can prevent you from making enough enzymes to digest food properly. When you're under stress and feeling anxious, your brain releases hormones to redirect your energy to your muscle, heart, and respiratory functions. Digestion takes a back seat when the body feels like it's facing an imminent safety threat. And yes, emotional trauma makes you feel threatened.

Chronic digestive issues that don't respond to strict nutrition protocols are usually rooted in brain-gut axis problems, and the main culprit in that arena is stress. Fearfulness, anxiety, and emotional trauma can impair the production of proteins that regulate peristalsis. When we're stressed out, our digestion is compromised. Prolonged patterns of stress, without our taking steps to manage and cope, can lead to brain-gut disorders like IBS and IBD. It's worth the time and effort to learn how to more efficiently manage stress, so it's not a major aggravator of your gut.

The Least You Need to Know

- Drugs such as painkillers, acid-reducers, and neutralizers, and even caffeine can disrupt stomach acid production and wreak havoc on your bowels.
- NSAIDs are a major contributor to the erosion of the stomach and intestinal wall and drastically increase your risk of bleeding ulcers.
- Antibiotics disrupt your gut microbiome and lead to dysbiosis and leaky gut.
- Alcohol abuse contributes to gut dysbiosis and intestinal hyperpermeability.
- Most of us have intestinal parasites, and if their populations are out of control they can lead to, or exacerbate, leaky gut and IBS symptoms.
- Stress can cause microbe imbalance in the gut and digestive distress.

Repairing the Leaks

Now you know the mechanics of your gut, what aggravates its processes, and what leads to digestive disease and intestinal hyperpermeability. Now you go about healing and sealing your gut lining.

Part 3 shows you the basics of how to repair the leaks in your gut lining that contribute to autoimmunity, food allergies, and inflammatory responses. We break down the process of identifying your symptoms and narrowing down the foods that trigger unwanted responses by using food diaries. You get an understanding of which foods and toxins are most likely to overburden your system, and we give you advice about how to flush your body of its toxic buildup and maintain your healthy gut with diet and stress management.

You learn how to introduce supplements and healthier options into your diet that will heal your gut. We share the guidelines from all the top nutrition experts on gut health, including the SCD, GAPS, and Paleo diets. You also learn how to implement meal planning strategies, brave the grocery store, conquer your kitchen, detox your home, and get ready for a healthy gut.

Healthy Gut Diet Basics

When people think "diet," too often they think about weight loss and sacrificing pleasurable experiences. Words have emotional ideas and history tied to them, and unfortunately *diet* often gets a bad rap. The first three *diet* definitions in the dictionary have little to do with notions of restriction and sacrifice. They're about habits and prescription. *Diet* primarily refers to the food and drink you consume or a regular basis or for a specific reason.

When you think about diet, try to think in terms of benefits. Diet is about the nourishment we provide our bodies so that we have the energy and health to do the things we love with vitality. We've spent a lot of time focusing on what damages the gut because the reality is that there are so many environmental influences, including food, that take a toll on the health of the intestinal lining. But there's so much out there in the world of food, nutrition, and the great outdoors that sustains the gut.

In this chapter, we examine the first steps needed to prepare ourselves and truly take responsibility for our gut health. You learn the logistics of how to begin healing and sealing the gut lining to prevent further intestinal hyperpermeability. You receive advice about cleansing techniques that flush your

In This Chapter

- Removing problematic foods from your diet
- Determining if certain foods trigger negative symptoms
- Foods that help calm your gut and heal your intestinal lining
- Starting the detox process

body of toxins and prepare it for the microbiota-enhancing foods that will establish beneficial microbes. This will, ultimately, give your gut and immune system the fuel they need to function optimally.

To start your journey toward a healthy gut, we review the food triggers to steer clear of, and we give you some specific guidelines for tracking nutritional progress and other tools for success. And we address stress management to ensure that life's pressures don't sabotage your best healthy gut efforts.

How the Diet Works

The basics of the healthy gut diet aren't new or revolutionary. If anything, the overarching principles we endorse actually turn back the clock as far as cooking methods and food sources go. Our modern diets have strayed away from whole foods and wholesome, nourishing meal preparation.

> **GUT WISE**
>
> One in four Americans eat some kind of fast food every day. Americans buy 31 percent more prepackaged foods than fresh foods. In a 2012 poll of "average Americans," 52 percent of people said they felt doing their taxes was easier than figuring out how to eat healthy. We hope we can make it *much* easier for you than doing your taxes.

We're not suggesting a return to the Stone Age. We enjoy and appreciate modern culture and technology. However, we do feel that our industrial processes often sacrifice the integrity and nutrient density of foods, and that's not a sacrifice we're willing to make. The advice offered by the healthy gut diet has to meet two main criteria:

- Everything we put on or into our bodies and immediate environment should not harm healthy digestive system function.

- When we take something into our bodies, we need to consider the impact on our gut bacteria. They outnumber our cells 10 to 1, and our genes 100 to 1. Gut bacteria must be kept in balance to maintain physical and mental health.

With these two goals in mind, here are some diet guidelines:

- Return to older cooking methods and meals made from whole foods.

- Eat healthy fats from pasture-raised, grass-fed, or wild-caught animals, but do so in moderation.

- Eat nutrient-dense foods from a variety of plant sources to ensure the intake of phytonutrients vital for enzyme production.

- Avoid the refined sugars and grains in processed foods, and feed your microbiota probiotics.

- Avoid toxic substances that are detrimental to beneficial microbes and digestive health in general.

So let's look at how to get started!

Eliminate Triggers That Damage the Gut

We've examined foods, medications, and substances that trigger intestinal hyperpermeability and aggravate the digestive system. You have to be your own quality control manager. This is especially true of the foods you eat every day. By now, you understand that you are what you eat. If what you're eating is damaging your system, don't gum up the works. Try to psyche yourself up for the task and reassociate trigger foods with the discomfort or even more serious health problems they've caused you.

When we refer to a "trigger," we mean foods and substances that set off a chain reaction in your gut, causing symptoms that make you uncomfortable and have a negative impact on your ability to enjoy life. But it's often helpful to first start by evaluating where you stand right now to get an idea of where you're coming from and what might need to be eliminated right away.

 ASK THE EXPERTS

When afflicted by illness, first identify and remove all causes of disease, then establish conditions of health. If we remove the symptoms and leave the cause, we have done nothing but lull ourselves into a false sense of security as the alarm stops sounding and the fire rages on.

—Mark Houliff, PhD, CNC, FAAIM, DCCN, Consultative Health and Nutrition

To get an idea of what your possible triggers might be, take a good hard look at what you're really eating. Documenting what you take into your body is a helpful, and often eye-opening, practice. This means writing down everything you put into and on your body; that is, make a list of all beauty and personal-care products in addition to everything you eat. It's probably best to keep the list of foods separate from what you apply topically to the outside of your body. Later in this chapter, we discuss some specifics on how to keep a food diary, which will also help you identify food triggers. And to help you get started, we provide some samples of these types of body product and food diaries in Appendix C.

Toxins for beauty and personal-care products will be covered extensively in Chapter 12. For now, let's start with food.

If you regularly consume processed meats, fatty red meats, gluten, low-fat or nonfat dairy, anything containing hydrogenated oils, anything containing high fructose corn syrup, soda, processed foods, excessive alcohol and caffeine, white rice, white bread, or white pasta, you already have some possible triggers you can start eliminating. Remember, these common triggers are generally no good for anyone's health. Try to reassociate them with disease.

Eat Microbiota-Enhancing Foods

One easy way to jump-start gut health is to eat foods that naturally encourage the growth of the most beneficial bacteria in your gut. And those microorganisms have some food preferences. All of the foods on the possible trigger list above feed pathogenic bacteria that love to attach to your intestinal wall, preventing you from absorbing vital nutrients and damaging the gut lining.

> **ASK THE EXPERTS**
>
> Let food be thy medicine, thy medicine shall be thy food.
>
> —Hippocrates, 460 to 370 B.C.E., Greek physician

Eating with your gut microbiota in mind can ease stress on the digestive system, improve immunity, and help decrease intestinal permeability. Some plant-based foods rich in vitamins and minerals that beneficial bacteria love are: bananas, artichokes, broccoli, cabbage, kale, cauliflower, and berries. Fermented foods are a great way to incorporate probiotics that will feed the right balance of microbe populations in your gut. We give you some more details in Chapter 10 and show you how to make your own in Chapter 14. Great fermented foods to try are sauerkraut, kimchi, yogurt, kefir, and miso.

Detoxing and Calming Your Body

Detoxing is basically the process of changing your body chemistry and flushing out the harmful materials that have built up in your system over time. You're likely to go through some kind of *withdrawal* as you reduce the amount of unhealthy food in your diet. The severity of your detox symptoms will depend entirely on the level of toxicity in your body's systems as well as how drastically you change your diet. Rest assured however, that any discomfort you experience while detoxing will be short-lived. (We cover more details on what to expect during detox in Chapter 16.)

It sounds counterintuitive to hear a downside to healthy behavior, but it's true. Detoxing can cause negative symptoms. When people stop eating unhealthy foods, they sometimes experience headaches or feel tired, down, restless, and almost like they have the flu. The good news is that even in severe cases where someone has always lived on processed foods and soda, these symptoms rarely last more than 2 weeks. Consider all of the negative effects of unhealthy eating on your gut microbiota, your immune system, and your entire body. Weigh your options and then try your best to stick out the detox process.

Anything you can do to decrease your body's toxic load is a step toward better gut health. Detoxing frees up your overtaxed liver that can't keep up with a constant flow of antigens and environmental toxins, especially if you have a hyperpermeable gut leaking these substances into the rest of the body.

Methylation, Glutathione, and the Detox Process

We discussed methylation in Chapter 5. Methylation is a chemical exchange in the body that makes gene expression possible. Methylation involves passing along a carbon atom linked to three hydrogen atoms from one molecule to another. This happens billions of times per second in the body. It makes cell repair and detoxification possible.

We need the methylation process to create a vital molecule in our bodies that is a detoxing powerhouse. *Glutathione* is a molecular MVP. It's a powerful *antioxidant* that protects against cell damage by neutralizing *free radicals* and stopping cell damage. Free radicals are unstable molecules that bond to the nearest molecule they can by effectively stealing one of their electrons. This can start off a whole chain reaction of formerly stable molecules becoming free radicals, too, because everyone is missing an electron and needs to steal one from someone else to become stable again. This domino effect leads to disease and an acceleration of the aging process.

Antioxidants are stable even when a free radical steals one of their electrons. That's what makes them so special. They stop the negative chain reaction of oxidative stress. Glutathione is a very gifted antioxidant. We need to do everything we can to help this molecule work its magic. We can start by eliminating toxic substances from our diet and immediate environment and eating foods that boost our glutathione levels.

> **DEFINITION**
>
> **Glutathione** is a molecule in the body that helps enzymes work in body detoxification processes. It acts as an antioxidant and consists of a chain of three fatty acids: glutamic acid, cysteine, and glycine. An **antioxidant** is any substance that counteracts the negative effects of oxidation in living organisms. **Free radicals** are unstable molecules who bind to other molecules to gain stability. This process causes oxidative stress, which leads to abnormal cell activity and damage.

Glutathione is made up of fatty acids that contain sulfur. Because sulfur is literally sticky, other molecules stick to it, including free radicals, heavy metals like mercury and aluminum, and other toxins. These toxins are then flushed out of our bodies through bile and eventually through our stools. Glutathione is like a disposable sticky broom that cleans up toxic dust as is travels through the body. It even recycles other antioxidants, like Vitamin C and E, and replenishes its own levels if we're feeding our body well and making healthy lifestyle choices. If we have an overload of toxins in our body, however, even this sticky power broom can't do its job properly.

Your methylation processes need to be running smoothly in order to provide energy to cells and produce enough glutathione to properly assist in the detoxing process. Eliminating trigger foods, eating probiotic and gut-balancing foods, and decreasing toxins in your body will all help you begin healing your gut. You can boost your glutathione production by exercising moderately for 30 minutes a day and eating foods rich in the sulfur compounds and amino acids.

Foods rich in the precursors to glutathione include garlic, onions, cruciferous vegetables (broccoli, kale, collards, cabbage, cauliflower, and watercress), and bone broths (more on these in Chapters 11 and 14). Supplements that help boost glutathione levels include vitamins C, E, B$_6$, and B$_{12}$ and the mineral selenium; folate (superior to the synthetic folic acid); milk thistle; N-acetylcysteine; and alpha-lipoic acid.

Cleanses and "Neutral" Foods to Start Detox

If you can already gauge from your past habits and exposure that your toxic load is pretty high and you're motivated to change, you might be tempted to engage in a drastic cleanse to jump-start your own detox process. A cleanse in this sense means to engage in a process that accelerates the elimination of toxins from the body. There are many fad cleanses and dramatic clinical cleanses available. We urge you to consult with a functional medicine or integrative health practitioner before undergoing any kind of invasive cleanse. The fact is that there are many more gentle cleansing activities involving time-tested methods and natural foods. We examine some of your options so you can make the best decision for yourself.

Enemas and colonics are popular cleansing techniques that can clear your colon of old fecal matter and toxins like candida and boost the overall detoxification process. If you suffer from heart, kidney, liver, or colon disease, you *should not* undergo either of these cleanses unless under the direct recommendation and supervision of a medical doctor. The colon retains and absorbs a lot of water during both enemas and colonics. This water retention can cause abnormal growths in the colon to bleed or rupture. Water absorbed during these procedures can also strain other diseased organs.

Enemas have been common home remedies for thousands of years and are useful for constipation as well as cleansing. They involve inserting a tube into the anus, which allows water or a mixture of water and another substance into the colon. You can purchase a kit over the counter at a pharmacy to safely administer an enema at home. Simply follow the instructions on the kit, hold the solution in for several minutes, and then evacuate the water solution into the toilet. You can add small amounts of chamomile or the contents of a probiotics capsule to the enema water beforehand, but only add what you would ingest orally. Probiotic enemas are an easy way to help repopulate the good gut bacteria at the same time you cleanse your colon and decrease your toxic load.

Colonics are performed at some doctors' offices, colonic hydrotherapy clinics, and wellness centers. Colonics take longer than enemas and involve a lot more water and can be dangerous if not administered correctly, so looking for a doctor who performs them is your safest bet.

An important thing to keep in mind with enemas and colonics is that performing them too often can lead to complications even worse than the symptoms you're trying to relieve. You have to be careful not to injure your colon wall if performing an enema yourself. If either of these cleanses is conducted often you can suffer from electrolyte imbalances and dehydration. Enemas and colonics should only be used on rare occasions to jump-start a detox, but after that rely on ingesting probiotics, eating healthy whole foods, and exercising regularly.

Another cleanse that flushes the colon from the inside, is to abstain from food for a few days and drink only water and a naturally cleansing juice that flushes your system. These types of cleanses can naturally detox your body and prepare your system for a healthier diet. Cleanses like this need to be done under the supervision of a dietitian who can gauge whether or not you're healthy enough for the challenges these methods can present. Performing a fast and liquid cleanse can have negative side effects. It's not for everyone.

YOU ARE WHAT YOU EAT

From 4 A.M. to 10 A.M., most people's bodies are in a natural detox mode. Eating a huge meal early in the morning can impede this process. (One more reason to celebrate the concept of brunch.) The best thing you can have first thing in the morning to help your daily detox is fresh fruit, water, freshly pressed juices, and probiotic-rich foods like yogurt. Juicing is especially effective first thing in the morning on an empty stomach.

Drinking fresh-pressed vegetable and fruit juices in conjunction with healthy, whole foods is an excellent way to boost your overall nutrient intake and health. Cleansing juices, however, are part of a more specialized short-term protocol (a dietary plan designed for healing). If you choose a fasting and juicing detox, it's most effective when you prepare your body a week ahead of time by cutting out all processed foods. Then for a few days (when you preferably have a long weekend and nothing much scheduled) you drink nothing but water interspersed with a few servings of juices.

Cayenne Lemonade Cleansing Juice

Here's a popular cleansing juice whose detoxing powers come from citrus and spice.

$\frac{1}{4}$ to $\frac{1}{2}$ tsp. cayenne, or to taste

4 TB. fresh lemon juice from an organic lemon

10 oz. warm filtered water (warm on the stove, not in a microwave to avoid "hot spots")

$\frac{1}{2}$ to 1 tsp. organic maple syrup or honey

1. Mix cayenne, lemon juice, water, and maple syrup in a blender.

2. Drink on an empty stomach.

GUT WISE

Don't be surprised if you feel the need to go to the bathroom pretty quickly. The drink is meant to stimulate your metabolism and jump-start the detoxing process.

Refreshing Apple Ginger Cleanse

This cleansing juice combines the medicinal powers of ginger and psyllium husk.

8 oz. fresh organic apple juice

1 tsp. ground ginger

1 tsp. psyllium husk

1. Mix apple juice, ginger, and psyllium husk in a blender.

2. Drink on an empty stomach.

These types of cleanses are short-term protocols (2 or 3 days) for people who may have a build-up of toxins and leaky gut but are not diabetic, hypoglycemic, or do not have heart disease. During a juice cleanse, it's important not to exercise or engage in any strenuous activity. After you finish a juice cleanse, it's important to slowly introduce calming and easy to digest foods such as watermelon and broths during the first day off the regimen. Then you can slowly add more complex solids like eggs and avocados, and start your well-balanced healthy diet, beginning with some "neutral" foods that will continue to cleanse your body while providing nourishment.

Some people want the benefits of a juice cleanse but find themselves too weak while trying to complete them. If you feel weak on a cleanse, stop the regimen and begin broths and then move back to solid foods. Some people find that they can better tolerate the cleanse with just one solid foods meal a day at lunchtime. Choose what feels best for you and always ask a dietitian for advice.

The following foods have the right balance of fiber and nutrients to work with your body while you're starting your healthy gut diet and detoxing your mind, body, and home:

- **Vegetables:** seaweed, broccoli, green beans, squash, carrots, beets, onions, garlic, celery, cucumber, artichokes, watercress, and asparagus

- **Fruits:** avocados, berries, lemons, limes, and grapefruit (Citrus in moderation.)

- **Animal proteins:** salmon, organic chicken, eggs, bone broths, and yogurt (Yogurt in moderation until you know it's not causing excess gas.)

You can even enjoy the benefits of a juicing detox while you enjoy the nourishment and satisfaction of real food. You don't have to stay on this limited diet for long, just the first several days (or the first several days after you perform a juice cleanse if you decide to do so under the consultation of a dietitian or integrative practitioner).

You can have produce raw or cooked. When you cook vegetables or meats, use full fat butter, unrefined virgin coconut oil, or ghee (a clarified butter that is pure milk fat without the casein proteins or lactose sugars that generally cause problems with dairy), and sauté or pan sear your foods instead of frying them.

Drinking a cup of green tea is okay while you're on this introduction diet. Other beverages that will be kind to your stomach while you're transitioning to this nutrition regimen are freshly juiced fruits and vegetables, ginger tea, almond milk, cashew milk, hemp milk, and coconut water. Salads dressed with room temperature olive oil, lemon juice, and spices are delicious. Other spices that will boost your detox efforts are fennel, ginger, and turmeric.

Stress Management

Stress management is critical to our health. We've looked at many ways in which the gut and the brain communicate and interact with one another. If you're not managing stress in some productive way, all of your nutritional efforts could be in vain. You'll still be sending those fight or flight hormones to the gut, and those microbiota will react to those messages. Finding a way to carve out some peace and quiet for yourself is a gift you give to your gut, your soul, and everyone around you. The less stressed you are, the more energy you'll have to devote to what's really important to you.

Meditation

Meditation is one way people find relief from stress. It's not just about structured techniques where everyone is sitting crossed-legged on the floor and chanting—although that's fine, too. The goal of any type of meditation is quieting your mind, acknowledging tension, consciously letting it go, and finding a sense of peace.

> **GUT WISE**
>
> In 2014, scientific studies at the University of Wisconsin in Madison have revealed that meditation can influence our genes, specifically the genes that modulate inflammatory responses. The RIPK2 and COX-2 genes that control inflammation are much less active in people who practice mindful meditation.

Research conducted at Harvard Medical School several years ago involved taking MRIs of participants' brains before and after an 8-week guided meditation program. They discovered that meditation actually changed structures in the brain. After 8 weeks of meditating for about 30 minutes a day, there was an increase in their gray matter in the part of the brain that controls self-awareness, introspection, and compassion. There was also a decrease of gray matter in the part of the brain in charge of anxiety and stress.

But you don't need intensive guided meditation classes to see results. Brief and effective meditations can be accomplished by just taking a few quiet moments at your desk to close your eyes and focus on your breathing while you mentally take stock of how you're feeling in your body at that moment. Wherever you feel tension, try to relax those muscles. You'll be surprised at how much you might be holding a tense posture or clenching your teeth or feeling stress in other areas of your body. Meditation is about allocating time to be present in the moment; scan your body for signs of stress, recognize that stress, and then relax into a more peaceful and calm state of mind.

Sleep

Sleep is paramount to our well-being. Science still doesn't understand the exact connection between sleep and the immune system, but the more sleep-deprived you are, the more your defenses are down. This leaves your gut and the rest of your body vulnerable to infections. Try your best to get at least 7 or 8 hours a sleep every night. When you're well-rested, the challenges of daily life and trying to attain your health goals won't seem as daunting. You need to recharge your mental and physical batteries with sleep.

> **GUT WISE**
>
> We've always known that a lack of sleep will make us irritable and confused, but we're just beginning to understand why. A study released in 2013 by the University of Rochester, New York, found that brain cells shrink while we sleep, allowing fluid to wash away by-products from around the cells more readily before sending them off to the liver for detoxification. When we're awake, the space between those same cells is dramatically restricted. It's as if our brains need us to be asleep for the clean-up crew to arrive. Sleep is part of our body's detox process, and we're just beginning to learn the mechanisms that make it possible.

Relaxation

Finding ways to carve out relaxing downtime are important. Just a quiet 5 minutes staring out the window can relieve stress. Sometimes, however, we need a little bit more than these 5-minute stress vacations. If you can afford a good Swedish or deep tissue massage, this kind of body-work can help boost your detox efforts as well as relieve tension. Just be sure it's with a licensed therapist and that you drink a lot of water after the massage. Deep tissue massages can release built-up toxins that were stored in the body. Drinking lots of water will help flush them out of your system.

There are plenty of free or low-cost ways to relieve stress and give yourself a mental break. One easy way to decompress and detox at the same time is a good-old-fashioned hot bath. Instead of pouring in bath oils or bubbles that might contain questionable ingredients, opt for DIY baths that soothe tired muscles and help draw body toxins out through the skin. Add 1 cup of apple cider vinegar, baking soda, seaweed powder, or Epsom salt to your bath water. Each of these ingredients has natural detoxing properties.

Exercise

Exercise is critical to overall health, and it's also a great stress management tool. You can channel your aggression or aggravation into a workout, and by the end of even a short session, you'll notice a reduction in tension. Exercise helps your GI tract, and it also helps your body release toxins and flush them out through your sweat. The endorphins it releases are excellent stress relievers, and they boost your mood.

ASK THE EXPERTS

A Certified Personal Trainer can help with your treatment through the therapeutic effects of exercise. The gastrointestinal tract is a muscle and should be treated as such. Just as the rest of your body's muscles are not getting use when you're sitting around all day, your GI tract doesn't either. Regular movement and moderate exercise can help "speed things along" and aid in digestion. However, too much jarring and too high of an intensity can have negative and unpleasant effects on a GI system. A personal trainer can develop a personalized exercise plan that will support to GI system and prevent negative side effects from overdoing it.

—Kristen Tice-Ziesmer, MS, RD, CSSD, LD, sports dietitian, ACE-Certified Personal Trainer, owner of Elite Nutrition and Performance

Identifying Problem Foods

You may already suspect you have food sensitivities because of your symptoms and your own research on them. Food diaries can help you track your personal symptoms and keep tabs on what you ate and when, so you can try to connect the dots for yourself. And your health-care practitioner can perform blood tests (such as the immunoglobulin panels discussed in Chapter 4 and later in this chapter), which will more accurately pinpoint what causes inflammation and allergic responses in your body, including food.

You can start by eliminating the list of common triggers we suggested earlier in this chapter. None of them are good for you or rich in necessary nutrients. If you really want to eat them in small to moderate amounts, it will at least help to know if your system can tolerate them. We give you suggestions for how to determine your personal food triggers in the later "Keep a Food Diary" section.

The IgG, IgE, IgM, and IgA Panels

Ask your dietitian, gastroenterologist, or integrative health practitioner to administer a full immunoglobulin bloodwork panel (see Chapter 4 for more information). The results can often reveal if top specific trigger foods like dairy and gluten are causing your immune system to go into overdrive—a very good sign that you're fighting a case of leaky gut syndrome.

Please note, however, that while these immunoglobulin tests are helpful, they have limitations. Sometimes antibodies, especially IgE antibodies, may be undetected by the test, or you may have antibodies that are responding to an antigen that is only present in processed food and the test panels only detect specific antigens in their original forms. You might only launch an immune response to a food once it's been chemically altered or cooked at high heat. The blood tests don't imitate those exact circumstances. This is just one more reason why you shouldn't eat processed foods.

Keep a Food Diary

In addition to any bloodwork you have performed, it's also wise that you take the initiative to keep a food diary. Ideally, you should keep a food diary of what you were eating before you made the commitment to a healthy gut and then one for when you begin your new diet. The first will give you a baseline for your old habits, so you have an honest view of what your toxic load might really be like.

A "before" food diary will also give you a real list of triggers to start eliminating. After you eliminate triggers, you can track any detox sickness you might feel as well as positive progress you're making. For example, you might notice that headaches you usually "fixed" with lots of coffee got even worse for 3 days after giving up caffeine, but then after that they went away for an entire week. You might also notice that you felt sluggish after giving up your sugary breakfast cereal, but that after the fourth day you felt like you had more energy in the morning.

To figure out your personal triggers, go on the neutral foods diet we suggested earlier in the chapter for a week or two. Then use a food diary to keep track of each trigger you try. Record when you ate a trigger food and how you felt in response to the food over the course of hours and days. (See Chapter 6 for a list of common trigger foods.) In this way, you can determine which foods are problematic. If you try to have dairy and gluten in the same meal, or even in the same day, and notice stomach pain or swelling in your joints a few hours later, you won't know which trigger caused it.

Only eat one trigger at a time for one week. For example, try only a single serving of dairy, like a small cup of yogurt, per day for a week. The next week you could try a slice of whole-wheat toast per day for a week. Record. Monitor. Wait. Evaluate. Repeat. (We show you how to conduct a skin sensitivity test before you even introduce triggers to help predict problematic foods in Chapter 17.)

Keeping a food diary is one of the harder parts of the diet because it involves a level of consistency that our busy lives can derail. But not if you make it easy for yourself. Use your smartphone or a notebook you keep with you at all times.

If you're looking for ultraconvenience and attention to detail, well, there's an app for everything these days. Let technology serve your best interests. Some outstanding tools are available online and for your smartphone that make keeping track of your nutritional information easier than ever. They all have free and paid features, so you can decide what's best and convenient for you. They're basically a way to make your food diary a digital and highly portable option. A lot of them even have online forums where you can message other members and forge your own network of virtual support to encourage each other and share information. Popular apps include My Fitness Pal, SparkPeople, and Cron-o-Meter. Check them out for yourself and see what works best for you.

Whether you decide to go old-school with a pencil and paper or opt for the high-tech versions, there are some things you need to keep in mind when logging your entries in a food diary:

- Be sure you include the date, time, and location of each food (i.e., you may find you can tolerate potatoes you cook at home but not cooked at a restaurant)

- Keep track of your symptoms on the same log as your food, and record the exact time you noticed them to make connections easier.

- Don't forget to list skin, joint, muscle, respiratory, energy levels, and even mood-related symptoms in addition to digestive symptoms.

- Record anything out of the ordinary, like headaches and feelings of anxiety. Some of these symptoms might be triggered by influences other than food, but it's better to have as much information as possible.

A food diary can help you do some detective work in figuring out your personal symptoms triggers, but it's also an amazing resource for a trained dietitian. Handing your findings to an integrative health practitioner will give them detailed data on your eating habits. Their professional eyes will spot patterns and connections you might miss.

Together, you and your dietitian can formulate an individualized plan for a healthy gut protocol that avoids negative food responses, and then carefully reintroduces triggers once the gut is healed and sealed. There are some triggers, such as refined sugar and grains, you should always avoid. But if some of your trigger foods have gut health benefits, like fermented dairy, eggs, and meats, you may want to reintroduce them eventually. Careful record-keeping will set you up for healthy gut success. We cover some more details about how to track your food intake, supplements, exercise, sleep habits, and stress levels in Chapter 17.

The Least You Need to Know

- Processed foods, gluten, dairy, and refined sugars are some of the most common culprits of intestinal hyperpermeability and compromised gut health.
- Eliminate common triggers from your diet and eat plenty of nutrient-dense fruits and vegetables and probiotic-rich fermented foods.
- Boost your detox processes by supporting glutathione levels in the body with vitamins C, E, B_6, B_{12}, folate, N-acetylcysteine, and alpha-lipoic acid.
- Juicing, fasting, and eating "neutral" foods can help calm and detox the body, preparing it for a healthy gut protocol.
- Manage stress and generate energy with exercise, meditation, and relaxation.
- In addition to immunoglobulin panels, keep a thorough food diary to track what you eat and any symptoms you notice after eating.

CHAPTER 10

Other Diet Plans

We're bombarded with a lot of nutritional advice in the media, online, and in popular culture in general. It's difficult to sort through the information and separate science from fads. The sensational claims of weight-loss diets and supplement companies add to the confusion about what constitutes healthy eating.

We selected the top nutritional advice from experts who gleaned their conclusions based on sound science with nutrient-dense eating and digestive health in mind. These diets aren't about counting calories; however, you'll probably lose any extra weight you've been carrying around, as all of these diets focus on sound nutrition and digestive health. A healthy body weight is the natural result of a healthy gut.

In this chapter, you learn the science and reasoning behind each major method. You understand why a method endorses or rejects certain foods based on how those foods most likely affect digestion and the gut microbiome. We also examine how the principles of each protocol contribute to a healthy gut.

In This Chapter

- The Specific Carbohydrate Diet guidelines and GAPS diet
- The premise behind the Paleo diet
- The argument for the low-FODMAP diet
- An overview of the Body Ecology Diet
- Benefits of the anti-inflammatory diet
- Principles of vegan and "nutritarian" approaches

The Specific Carbohydrate Diet (SCD)

Dr. Sidney Valentine Haas (1870–1964) developed the Specific Carbohydrate Diet (SCD) to treat celiac disease, which in the days of Dr. Haas's practice, was not as clearly defined as it is today. The term *celiac* used to include a wide range of IBS-type digestive problems. Once celiac was identified as an autoimmunity triggered by gluten (or *gluten-induced enteropathy*), the diet was largely forgotten by medicine, and celiac disease was treated with a gluten-free diet. But simply ditching gluten didn't help everyone who had previously fallen under that much larger "celiac" umbrella.

The mother of one of Dr. Haas's patients, Elaine Gottschall, had not forgotten what his treatments had done for her little girl in 1958. Gottschall brought her daughter to Dr. Haas in the hopes his nutrition protocol would help her child who had ulcerative colitis coupled with neurological symptoms. After 2 years on the SCD, the girl was symptom free. Gottschall, who was also a biochemist, spent years helping others experience similar results. In 1987, she popularized Dr. Haas's approaches in her book *Breaking the Vicious Cycle: Intestinal Health Through Diet.*

Dr. Sydney Haas's Main Principles of SCD

Dr. Hass recommended the elimination of *disaccharide* and *polysaccharide* sugars. These types of sugars, that are in essence carbohydrates, are difficult for a lot of us to break down into simple sugars, which are more easily absorbed by the body. Disaccharides are often called "double sugars" because they contain two simple sugars joined together. Disaccharides include sucrose (table sugar and the sugar naturally occurring in sugar cane and fruits), lactose (milk sugar), and maltose (found in molasses and formed when starch digests). Polysaccharides include cellulose (found in plants), starch (found in vegetables), and pectin (found in fruits and some grains and legumes).

DEFINITION

Gluten-induced enteropathy is another term for celiac disease. If you have celiac disease, ingesting gluten causes small intestinal inflammation, excessive zonulin production, and therefore a hyperpermeable intestinal lining. Left untreated, this condition leads to chronic diarrhea, weight-loss, and malnutrition. A **disaccharide** sugar is made up of two simple sugars (monosaccharides) joined together in a chemical bond in which one molecule of water is removed. **Polysaccharides** are comprised of longer chains of three or more monosaccharides.

The SCD seems restrictive at first glance because it doesn't allow complex carbs or most starchy vegetables. But it does encourage eating lots of nonstarchy vegetables, ripened fruit, animal proteins and fats, and lactose-free dairy. Most full-fat fermented dairy is virtually lactose-free because the bacteria consume the lactose during the fermenting process. There are also some aged cheeses with tiny amounts of lactose that are permitted on the diet.

Here's an overview of some of the foods on the "Do eat" and "Do not eat" lists for the first 6 months of the SCD diet:

Do eat:

- Animal proteins, including eggs and all nonprocessed meats that are grass-fed, free ranging, and antibiotic free.

- Plant-based proteins in their natural state (or as a "butter" with no additives,) such as almonds, Brazil nuts, cashews, chestnuts, pecans, hazelnuts, walnuts, peanuts, white beans, navy beans, lentils, split peas, lima beans, kidney beans, and black beans.

- Fresh or frozen vegetables, such as asparagus, beets, broccoli, brussels sprouts, cabbage, cauliflower, carrots, celery, cucumbers, eggplant, garlic, kale, lettuce, mushrooms, onions, peas, peppers, pumpkin, spinach, squash, string beans, tomatoes, and watercress.

- Ripe fresh or frozen fruits, such as apples, avocados, bananas, berries, coconuts, dates, grapefruit, grapes, kiwis, kumquats, limes, mangoes, melons, nectarines, oranges, papayas, peaches, pears, pineapples, prunes, raisins, rhubarb, and tangerines.

- Dairy, such as organic full-fat fermented yogurt, 30-day aged cow and goat cheeses from organic sources, full-fat butter, ghee, and dry-curd cottage cheese.

- Spices are allowed in their natural states. If a prepared mix of spices is used, make sure there are no anti-caking agents added. (These often have added chemicals and even gluten in them.)

- Beverages, such as weak coffee or tea in moderation, water, club soda, freshly pressed fruit and vegetable juices in moderation, and selected alcohol (dry wine, gin, rye, scotch, bourbon, and vodka) also in moderation.

- Honey is the only approved sweetener.

Take note of how many things you *can* eat on this plan. It's really about eliminating some of the major triggers we've already covered, which is demonstrated by this next list.

Do not eat:

- Processed proteins, such as ham, processed sausages (which included hot dogs and other meat "dogs," luncheon meats, and bratwurst).

- The following legumes: soybeans, chickpeas, bean sprouts, mung beans, and fava beans.

- The following vegetables: corn, all vegetables in the tuber family (potatoes, yams, sweet potatoes, arrowroot, parsnips, and turnips), any canned vegetables (unless they are organic and contain no additives), and starch powders derived from vegetable starches (cornstarch, arrowroot, and tapioca).

- Canned fruit (unless it's organic with no additives) or commercially processed fruit juices.

- No grains are allowed, this includes wheat, barley, rye, oats, rice, buckwheat, millet, triticale, bulgur, spelt, and quinoa.

- None of the following dairy: milks or creams of any kind, commercially produced yogurt, nonorganic cheeses and cheese products, regular curd cottage cheese, feta, mozzarella, and ricotta.

Whew! That's some list. While it's extensive, we felt it was important to include because so many other diets purported to heal and seal the gut build upon the science that backs the Specific Carbohydrates Diet. Some of these foods can be gradually reintroduced into the diet after 6 months using a method like the one we discussed with the food diary in Chapter 9: one trigger at a time per week while carefully monitoring and recording symptoms. Individual tolerances for different foods will vary, but the preceding lists are guidelines for how to start.

Healing the Gut with the Right Carbs

The rationale for the inclusion and exclusion of the foods on the "do eat" and "do not eat" lists is based on being gentle to a damaged gut. Complex carbs and processed foods put a strain on our digestive system, and some of these substances injure the gut lining, compromise the integrity of the intestinal wall, and alter the composition of our gut microbiota.

GUT WISE

Without gut microbes we wouldn't be able to digest complex carbs at all. One more thing to thank them for.

Getting rid of the polysaccharides and most disaccharides that require more work to digest will give an overtaxed gut time to heal. Without these carbohydrates in the body, the microbiota populations can stabilize themselves. A balanced gut microbiome will communicate with the brain better, help us absorb nutrients better, and help our immune system function properly. Without processed foods, the toxic load in the body diminishes. As zonulin levels stabilize, tight junction function can return to normal levels and decrease the flood of antigens being released into the bloodstream. Less antigens means less inflammation in the gut and the entire body.

The GAPS Diet

GAPS stands for Gut and Psychology Syndrome. Dr. Natasha Campbell-McBride, the diet's architect, is a medical doctor who studied neurology and nutrition after her son was diagnosed with autism. She was determined to find the underlying causes of his condition.

The overarching goal of the GAPS nutritional protocol is to bring balance to the ecosystem in the gut to heal the intestinal wall. This approach aims to stop gut hyperpermeability in order to prevent toxins from overloading a person's immune system and to ensure proper nutrient absorption by healing the digestive tract.

Dr. Campbell-McBride recommends following her program for at least 2 years to make sure the gut heals and the entire body detoxes. This is accomplished by first detoxing and healing the GI tract and then working to detox the rest of the body's systems. Once the gut is healed and sealed, a person can gradually add other more commonly eaten foods into the diet, but it's recommended to never go back to eating processed foods again.

Dr. Natasha Campbell-McBride and the Expansion of the SCD

The nutrition protocols recommended in GAP rides the coattails of the SCD. And there are now even newer incarnations that piggyback on the principles of GAPS. Dr. Campbell-McBride is very forthcoming about having expanded and modified the SCD based on the outcomes she observed in her patients. While the SCD's main purpose is to calm an irritated digestive tract, GAPS also focuses on the entire brain-gut axis and correcting digestive, psychological, and cognitive disorders associated with disruptions in that axis.

GAPS emphasizes probiotic foods and supplementation that Campbell-McBride proposes may be a lifelong commitment, as some people's microbiota might revert easily to dysbiosis once the influx of probiotics stops. Another expansion of the diet is the focus on the nutrient density and rate of absorption of foods. GAPS relies on bone broths and organ meats to remedy nutrient deficits and soothe and heal the gut lining.

The Link Between Diet and Learning Disabilities

Dr. Campbell-McBride is a staunch believer in the gut-brain axis connection and that pathogenic bacteria seeping into the bloodstream via a leaky gut contribute directly to learning disabilities. Processed sugars and grains are on her list of the biggest contributors to the inflammation running rampant in GAPS patients.

GAPS prescribes removing not just food triggers, but also environmental toxins. (We cover many of these toxins in Chapter 12.) The theory is that an overloaded liver and immune system choked with the constant influx of antigens is also inept at filtering out the noxious substances we're bombarded with in our personal care products and home cleaners. Furthermore, Dr. Campbell-McBride makes a case for how gluten and casein proteins, as well as toxic residue (from herbicides, pesticides, and other chemical exposure), actually cross the blood-brain barrier and interfere with normal brain function. With so many antigens, pathogens, and toxins flooding the system, cognitive disorders and learning disabilities become inevitable. GAPS aims to treat the entire brain-gut axis.

Foods to Avoid

A lot of foods need to be removed in the initial stages of the GAPS diet because the damaged gut lining cannot produce the needed enzymes to break down and absorb their nutrients properly. They will only ferment in the gut and feed pathogenic bacteria whose overgrowth continues to damage the gut lining. That would only lead to enterocytes that don't function properly, tight junctions that open too widely, antigens that enter the bloodstream, and the whole messy cycle would go on and on. The GAPS approach to stopping the cycle is to remove the food that feeds the undesirable bacteria and introduce foods that will repopulate the beneficial microbiota.

The "Do Not Eat" list for GAPS for the first several weeks is very similar to the SCD list. They both eliminate all processed foods, refined sugars, and complex carbs. GAPS prohibits *all* legumes for the first stage instead of a select few. The restrictions for dairy are stricter as well. There is no commercial dairy of any kind and only homemade ghee is allowed for the first 6 weeks and only if it doesn't cause a negative symptom for you. After 6 weeks, fermented dairy is allowed if you have no negative responses. This initial restriction takes into account the caseins in milk products, how easily they are absorbed by the brain, and how the wide range of antigens in milk products can make them a problem for the immune system in the gut and beyond.

YOU ARE WHAT YOU EAT

On the GAPS diet, fruit is best digested alone as a snack, or with nuts and seeds. It's recommended that fruit is not eaten with large meals. According to GAPS guidelines, meat of some kind needs to accompany every meal. Dr. Campbell-McBride's research suggests that fruit (with the exception of the avocado) can interfere with meat digestion. Fruit is also best eaten ripe to avoid as many of the complex carbs that are natural in fruit. The riper the fruit, the more these carbs break down before we eat them.

Best Foods to Eat

Here is an overview of the basic food recommendations for the first 6 weeks of the GAPS diet:

- Sweeten with honey only.

- Fruit must be eaten ripe.

- Only nonstarchy vegetables allowed. (See SCD vegetable guidelines.)

- Eggs, meat, and fish (as long as there are no preestablished allergies to these foods). Poach, boil, or stew because frying, roasting, and grilling make meats harder to digest.

- Bone broths are the beverage of choice with a meal. Water or other fluids during meals impede the production of digestive enzymes.

- Between meals, drink bone broth and freshly pressed juices and filtered water (especially water with sliced lemon or 1 teaspoon of apple cider vinegar containing the "mother"— Bragg's brand is readily available).

- Almond milk and coconut milk are allowed if they are homemade or organic-sourced with no additives beyond water and honey.

GUT WISE

The GAPS diet has some very specific instructions for introducing dairy. Some people can tolerate ghee from the very beginning. But if they can't, it's introduced with butter after 6 weeks of being on the first phase of the diet. Ghee and butter are both extremely low in lactose and casein. Before introducing either of them, conduct a skin sensitivity test. (See directions in Chapter 17). If there is a skin reaction, wait 6 weeks and try again. After tolerating ghee and butter for 6 weeks, introduce fermented dairy (homemade or organic). The microbes in the yogurt can then go to work repopulating the gut and helping bring balance to your microbiota.

After 6 weeks, dairy can slowly be introduced, and then after another period of 6 weeks, other whole-food former triggers can be introduced in the same manner we discussed earlier. It is still recommended that processed foods never be a part of your diet again. If your gut is especially leaky, you have multiple food allergies, an autoimmune condition, a learning disability, or a mood disorder, the GAPS guidelines prepare you for a long-haul approach with the diet that is very gradual and could take up to 2 years.

The Paleo Diet

The Paleolithic period of history lasted from roughly 2.5 million to 10,000 years ago. Our ancestors lived in an era without agriculture and certainly without industry, so they lived as hunter-gatherers. They foraged for fruit and tuber vegetables, hunted mammals, and eventually developed tools for fishing.

> **GUT WISE**
>
> The gut bacteria of the indigenous tribes of the Andes Mountains are 47 percent more diverse than those of the average American. They've been hunters and gatherers for 11,000 years.

There is a large body of research that suggests that our bodies haven't evolved to handle foods beyond those similar to the ones eaten by our ancestors. Cultivated grains, legumes, and dairy are off-limits according to the Paleo experts, because our bodies are not genetically programmed to digest them or derive nutrients from them.

Dr. Loren Cordain and the Paleo Premise

Dr. Loren Cordain holds a PhD in Health and is a professor of Health and Exercise at the Colorado State University. He has become something of a celebrity in the world of nutrition by espousing that optimal gut health and general well-being is best achieved by adhering to the diet of our Stone Age predecessors. He has extensively studied Paleolithic nutrition. Here's a breakdown of the major principles of the diet:

- Increase protein to around 19 to 35 percent of your calories, making meat, eggs, and seafood your staple foods.

- Carbs should be nonstarchy fresh fruits and vegetables with low glycemic indexes and high fiber content. Carbs should be 35 to 45 percent of daily calories.

- Your fat intake should be made up of mostly *monounsaturated* and *polyunsaturated fats* balanced with omega-3s and omega-6s. (We discuss omega-3s and omega-6s in detail in Chapter 11.)

- You need to have a balance of acid-producing foods (meat, fish, and salt) and *alkaline* foods (fruits and vegetables) for optimal kidney, bone, and respiratory health.

These principles govern what is encouraged and what is off-limits for Paleo eaters.

> **DEFINITION**
>
> **Monounsaturated fats** contain only one double bond in each of their molecules and are associated with lower "bad" LDL cholesterol. **Polyunsaturated fats** have two or more double bonds in their molecules and are present in nuts, seeds, fish, algae, and leafy greens. **Alkaline** compounds have a pH greater than seven and are capable of neutralizing acids.

The Paleo Hunter-Gatherer Guidelines

Here are the general foods allowed and restricted for modern Stone Age eaters.

Do eat:

- Grass-fed and free-range meats, eggs, and seafood

- Fruits and nonstarchy vegetables

- Nuts and seeds

- Healthy oils, such as olive, walnut, avocado, coconut, and flaxseed

Do not eat:

- Grains of any kind

- Legumes of any kind (including peanuts)

- Dairy of any kind

- Refined sugars, oils, and processed foods

- Tuber vegetables, such as potatoes

- Table salt

There is some overlap of agreement between the SCD, GAPS and the Paleo diet, but note the absence of dairy and all legumes in the Paleo diet.

> **YOU ARE WHAT YOU EAT**
>
> There is a lot of praise in the Paleo, SCD, and GAPS literature for organ meats and their nutritional density. And the superstar of organ meats is liver. If you suffer from anemia, liver is a must to help you recover.

There is no "introductory period" or "weaning off" period for trigger foods on the Paleo diet. You simply don't consume any foods that would typically cause a problem in most people with intolerances and leaky gut symptoms. There is no fermented dairy to provide those wonderful probiotics, but probiotic supplements, fermented vegetables, and coconut milk yogurt are allowed.

The Body Ecology Diet

Like the GAPS diet, the Body Ecology (BE) Diet focuses primarily on balancing the gut microbiome and detoxing the body. The major difference between the two diets is in how the Body Ecology Diet addresses how to clear the body of a pathogenic candida problem.

The founder of the Body Ecology Diet, Donna Gates, and Dr. Campbell-McBride have lectured together and have professional respect for one another. They have each leaned heavily on each another's research to improve their approaches: Gates for Dr. Campbell-McBride's explanation of the brain-gut axis connection to psychological and cognitive disorders, and Dr. Campbell-McBride for Gates' inclusion and reliance on fermented foods as the primary source of probiotics in a healthy gut protocol.

Donna Gates, MEd, ABAAHP, and the BE Premise

Donna Gates is a nutritionist and anti-aging medical practitioner who devised a diet free of sugar, gluten, and casein that is rich in fermented foods and probiotics. The main premise of the Body Ecology Diet is that it will heal the inner ecosystem of the microbiome and promote digestive and immune health.

Along with the diet come many suggested supplements for detoxing and promoting beneficial gut bacteria populations. The diet is also comprised of three phases. In Phase 1, fermented vegetables and kefir made from coconut water are added. In Phase 2, you eliminate processed foods, fatty red meats, and trans fats, and introduce natural oils and organic free-range meats. In Phase 3, you reduce your carbs and sugars by cutting out grains, potatoes, and most fruits. Later on, you can slowly increase your intake of some of the foods phased out in the last stage.

BE Dietary Guidelines

The "dos" and "don'ts" of the BE diet are more restrictive than anything we've looked at so far. Additionally, the regimen encourages the use of multiple supplements promoted by the diet founder, and many of them are very expensive.

Do eat:

- Fermented vegetables

- Yogurt and kefir made with coconut water

- Healthy oils: flaxseed, olive oil, and coconut oil

- Organic eggs

- Seafood

- Organic grass-fed and free-range lean meats

- Seeds

- Limited grains and seeds (after you've completed all three phases), such as quinoa, amaranth, millet, and buckwheat

Do not eat:

- Gluten

- Dairy

- Refined sugars and all processed foods

- Fatty meats or any nonorganic commercially farmed meats

Of all the diets we've looked at so far, this one is by far the most restrictive. You'll have to decide for yourself if the benefits outweigh the drawbacks.

The Low-FODMAP Diet

If you suffer from IBS symptoms or IBD, and your digestive distress is your primary concern above all others, you should take a close look at the low-FODMAP diet. FODMAPs is an acronym for fermentable *oligosaccharides,* disaccharides, monosaccharides, and *polyols.* These substances are short-chain carbohydrates that cause problems for IBS and IBD sufferers. They aren't absorbed well in the intestine, and some individuals are really sensitive to the extra work it takes for the digestive system to break down these suckers. The end result in sensitive guts is microbiota working overtime to ferment the leftovers. The gas produced during the fermentation process can create painful symptoms.

> ***DEFINITION**
>
> **Oligosaccharides** are carbohydrates whose molecules are generally made up of between 3 and 10 monosaccharides. Oligosaccharides are often referred to as a prebiotic food for bacteria. **Polyols** are carbohydrates whose molecular structure is similar to both sugar and alcohol, which is why they're often referred to as "sugar alcohols." Polyols are used as sweeteners and include sorbitol, mannitol, and xylitol.

The goal of the FODMAPs diet is to remove the short-chain carbs from the diet completely, give the gut bacteria a break from all the fermenting, and give you a break from all the pain and discomfort that process causes. After several weeks, FODMAPs are then gradually reintroduced in small amounts.

Implement a Low-FODMAP Diet

With a 74 percent success rate, if you suffer from IBS or IBD, this diet is worth a try. Eliminating the food bacteria ferment is the first major step in the diet. No fermenting also means less bacteria waste products swimming around in your system. Too much of that stuff can cause pressure in our gut, leading to stomach pain and acid reflux. Bacteria waste products can also promote diarrhea. So how do you get started to see if a low-FODMAP diet will ease your symptoms? Don't eat foods high in FODMAPs.

To implement the diet, cut out the following foods for 4 to 6 weeks:

- Fruits: apple, apricot, avocado, blackberry, cherry, lychee, nectarine, peach, pear, persimmon, plum, prune, watermelon, and all dried fruit

- Vegetables: asparagus, artichoke, beetroot, bell pepper, broccoli, brussels sprouts, cabbage, cauliflower, eggplant, fennel, garlic, leek, mushroom, okra, onion, shallot, and sweet corn

- All legumes (including all types of beans)

- All dairy

- Grains: wheat, rye, barley (basically all gluten)

- Sweeteners: honey, corn syrup, sorbitol, mannitol, xylitol, isomalt, and maltitol

It's important to keep a food diary for the 4- to 6-week period to track your symptoms or lack of symptoms. That "lack" is what we're going for!

Wean Off of Low FODMAPs

After a 4- to 6-week period without FODMAPs in your diet, you're hopefully feeling great and not experiencing uncomfortable gas, bloating, heartburn, or diarrhea. You've eliminated a source of stress and inflammation for your digestive system and given your microbiota a chance to rebalance themselves. Maybe some SIBO you had going on with all those extra carbs to eat and ferment has subsided. This is when you test the waters and reintroduce one FODMAP food at a time, waiting at least several days between each food.

Most people find this break from high FODMAPs was all they needed to reboot their systems, but you have to tread carefully to find out. Keeping a food diary is paramount to the success of this diet. You need to track not only what you ate and when you ate, but how much. Record your exact portion.

You might find you have a threshold for how much of a certain FODMAP-containing food you can eat. This level of tolerance is very personal, and a food diary is an excellent tool to help you track that tolerance. You may find that one small serving of broccoli is all you can handle without bloating and gas. Again, like other diets we're examining, it will take some perseverance and personal detective work and adjustment to find the portions and combinations of food your gut likes best.

If you've tried other protocols first and still suffer from bloating and diarrhea specifically, low FODMAPs could prove very helpful. Unlike the other diets we've look at, low FODMAPs doesn't tout itself as a cure for anything. It's meant to be a short-term cleanse and reintroduction method with reasonable limits. FODMAP foods in moderation are good for us due to their prebiotic effects. Your beneficial bacteria need the food, but just like us, sometimes too much of a good thing leads to disaster.

The Anti-Inflammatory Diet

Inflammation is part of our immune system's response. The white blood cell rally call is heard throughout the body, bringing swelling, heat, and more immune cells to the site of infection and injury. But intestinal hyperpermeability leaks antigens into our system and causes immune system overdrive. When inflammation isn't working to stop an infection or promote healing, it damages healthy tissues.

We've examined many root causes of inflammation, especially inflammation as a result of auto-immunity. Genes and environment play a role, but we know from epigenetics that we can control some factors that influence gene expression. Good nutrition is the cornerstone of fighting unnecessary inflammation in the body. This is the premise of the anti-inflammatory diet.

Premise and Major Proponent, Integrative Medicine Pioneer Dr. Andrew Weil

Dr. Andrew Weil is one of the most famous and influential integrative practitioners of our time. Before obtaining his medical degree from Harvard, he earned an undergraduate degree in botany (also from Harvard). Dr. Weil certainly applies his knowledge of plants in his practices today. He is the founder and director of the Arizona Center for Integrative Medicine at the University of Arizona.

As a kind of poster child for integrative medicine, Dr. Weil has paid a lot of public relations dues in the media to shed light on complementary and alternative medicine. As an open-minded medical doctor, his philosophy is to follow conventional medical advice and supplement with alternative therapies. Sound nutrition, however, does not constitute an alternative; it's the foundation for good health. His general tips are to eat a wide variety of the freshest foods possible, eat plenty of colorful fruits and vegetables for vital *phytonutrients,* and avoid processed and fast food.

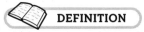 **DEFINITION**

Phytonutrients are substances found in certain plants that promote health and may even prevent disease.

Anti-Inflammatory Diet Guidelines

Dr. Weil has some specific guidelines about the distribution of calories in the ideal diet, and he doesn't restrict the same trigger foods as the other protocols. A basic meal should include carbs, fat, and protein, and the distribution of your daily calories should be 40 to 50 percent carbs,

30 percent fat, and 20 to 30 percent protein. Aim for the lower side of the protein margins if you have an autoimmune condition or allergies as the source of inflammation in your body.

There isn't a strict "do eat" and "do not eat" list, but rather an attitude of "try to incorporate more _____" and "avoid _____."

The advice about carbs is to eat more squashes, cruciferous vegetables, beans (including soy), and whole grains, but avoid wheat and all processed foods and refined grains and sugars. You could even enjoy pasta on this diet if it's in moderation and cooked al dente.

Fats should be consumed at a ratio of 1:2:1—saturated to monounsaturated to polyunsaturated fat. Avoid all hydrogenated oils of any kind, including margarine and vegetable shortening. Suggested sources of healthy fats that are also proteins are walnuts, cashews, almonds, avocados, fatty fish like salmon, organic cheese, and yogurt. Fiber intake also needs to be higher than what most of us typically consume. Berries, vegetables, and whole grains are recommended sources.

Specific daily recommendations for how many grams of carbs, fats, and protein women and men should consume are based on the standard 2,000 calories a day.

Anti-Inflammatory Diet Daily Intake Recommendations

	Carbohydrates	Fat	Protein	Fiber
Men	240 to 300 grams	67 grams	80 to 120 grams	40 grams
Women	160 to 200 grams	67 grams	80 to 120 grams	40 grams

In addition to these specific dietary suggestions, Dr. Weil does suggest some supplements. Antioxidant supplements should be taken with the largest meal of the day and should include: 200 milligrams vitamin C, 400 IU vitamin E, 200 micrograms selenium, 10,000 to 15,000 IU mixed carotenoids, 400 micrograms folic acid, and 2,000 IU vitamin D. Some carotenoids help your body make vitamin A, and they are also powerful antioxidants. Menstruating women can also take iron supplements and 500 to 700 milligrams of calcium citrate daily. Other supplements include 2,000 to 3,000 milligrams of fish oil, 60 to 100 milligrams of coenzyme Q_{10}, and 100 to 400 milligrams of alpha-lipoic acid.

This is quite a list, but the overall impact is to protect your cells against damage, help natural detox processes, support the immune system, and prevent inflammation everywhere in the body, including the gut.

The Vegan and "Nutritarian" Approaches

While some of the diets we've examined so far encourage the use of bone broths and animal proteins, these approaches recommend limiting animal products to just fish and eggs, or even eliminating them altogether. Each diet has its own rationale for why animal proteins should be scaled down or ditched altogether. Philosophical and animal rights issues aside, there is some science that suggests animal proteins might not be for everyone. Let's investigate.

Veganism for a Healthy Gut?

A vegan diet is entirely plant-based with zero animal products. Plant protein and phytonutrients will help your body run smoother, including digestion. This is a fact, but the main danger in subtracting animal proteins is not having enough diversity. Vitamin B_{12} deficiency is also a major concern here. In a vegan diet, you have to supplement this crucial vitamin, as it doesn't exist in plant-based sources. Without enough vitamin B_{12}, you can develop nerve disorders and anemia.

There are some valid arguments for at least limiting animal products. Too much animal protein has been shown to spike levels of IGF-1, which is a substance similar to insulin in the body. Some studies show that elevated levels of IGF-1 can increase cancer risks and speed up the aging process in general. Red meat in particular has high concentrations of iron, which are beneficial, but the protein that carries the iron (called heme) can have a negative impact on gut health. Too much heme can damage the lining of our GI tract.

> **GUT WISE**
>
> Protein shakes and "fake meat" patties are very popular among vegetarians and vegans, but look at the ingredients carefully. Soy protein isolate is commonly used in meat-alternative products and is in around 60 percent of processed foods. The manufacturing of this ingredient requires aluminum, some of which remains in the finished product you eat. Aluminum has been linked to dementia and Alzheimer's disease.

Becoming a vegan will only contribute to gut health if you diversify your fruits and veggies, get complex carbs from gluten-free whole grains, take in protein from sources like nuts, legumes in moderation, and non-GMO fermented soy, and supplement with a broad-spectrum probiotic. Satisfying your hunger by overloading on processed flours and grains and white potatoes will spike your blood sugar and contribute to SIBO. Balance is key.

The Nutritarian Diet

Nutritarian is a term coined by medical doctor and nutrition expert Dr. Joel Fuhrman. His advice for gut health and general well-being is to eat all you want of low-calorie, nutrient-dense foods. Doing this over time will bring a person to a natural understanding of when they've met their caloric needs. We only suffer from food cravings when we eat junk that doesn't satisfy our body's nutrition needs.

In a nutritarian diet, there is no calorie counting, just whole foods, very limited animal products, and no processed foods. There is no consumption of anything that would overfeed the pathogenic bacteria. Overall, the diet promotes healthy GI function, outstanding immune system support, and general well-being.

According to Dr. Fuhrman, for optimal health animal products should comprise 10 percent or less of your total caloric intake. He recommends that portions of animal products should also be limited to 4 ounces or less and to avoid making animal protein the focus of the meal. One of the main rationales for limiting animal proteins is that they lack fiber, so they take longer to make their way through our digestive tracts. The caveat here is too make sure you know where your food is coming from and that it's not chock-full of antibiotics and pollutants.

 YOU ARE WHAT YOU EAT

> Fish is a healthy source of omega-3s and protein, but mercury contamination is a real concern. Mercury can block the absorption of nutrients and damage the mucous membranes in the GI tract. It interrupts the body's absorption of zinc, which contributes to immune function and the breakdown of carbohydrates. Mercury disrupts the body's natural mechanisms for filtering out toxic metals via the liver and kidneys. Fish low in mercury include flounder, scallops, trout, squid, and salmon. The highest mercury levels are found in swordfish, mackerel, tilefish, and shark. A complete list of fish mercury levels can be found at nrdc.org/health/effects/mercury/guide.asp.

The nutritarian approach to gut health is in essence about limiting animal protein, eating mostly gluten-free whole grains in moderation, and eating all the fruits and vegetables you want.

The Least You Need to Know

- The SCD diet eliminates complex carbs, gluten, lactose, and processed foods. The GAPS diet builds on this with detox measures, bone broths, and probiotics.

- The Paleo diet advocates a return to Stone Age hunter-gatherer nutrition, which is free of gluten, dairy, legumes, and processed foods.

- The low-FODMAP diet advises those with IBS or IBD to take a 6-week break from the fermentable short-chain carbs that are hard on the GI tract.

- The Body Ecology Diet cuts out sugars, gluten, casein, all processed foods, and supplements with detox aids and probiotics.

- The anti-inflammatory diet practices moderation of all whole foods groups, avoidance of processed foods, and supplementation of vitamin and mineral.

- Vegan diets eliminate all animal products while the nutritarian diet allows them in moderation and focuses on nutrient-dense plant foods.

Your Healthy Gut Diet Plan

In this chapter, you learn how to combine everything you've learned so far and apply it toward taking those first steps in the healthy gut diet. We distill the most sensible advice from top nutrition experts and give you an overview of the best steps to take toward reclaiming your digestive health.

You've already learned what your gut needs, now let's look at how to put all that knowledge into action.

In This Chapter

- A consensus of the best advice on achieving optimal gut health
- Trigger foods to remove from your diet
- Foods that restore your microbiota and heal the gut lining
- Cracking your own personal healthy gut code
- Healthy gut supplements

A Consensus for a Healthy Gut Diet

One of the cool things about you is that you picked up this book to learn about the engine that powers the human body. By now you've learned that it's a complicated beast of a machine with many parts and an entire other microscopic kingdom living inside of it that has its own needs and agenda. Who knew you were eating for two? (Although, it's really more like eating for several trillion.)

It would be simple if we were like cars, and all we needed was one kind of fuel. But you have trillions of cells in your body with enormously diverse functions. You also have trillions of microbiota living in there with those cells. You're a sophisticated part-human/part-bacterial being who needs a whole variety of fuels. Human/bacteria beasts are a little high-maintenance that way.

Here are some low-maintenance first steps to get your high-maintenance machine on track for a healthy gut diet:

- Start by cutting out casein, gluten, and all processed foods. (This includes white sugar, white rice, white bread, and table salt).

- Detox your body and home. (See tips in Chapter 9 for the body and Chapter 12 for the home.)

- Gradually introduce probiotics, fermented foods, and the supplements we suggest later in this chapter.

- Eat lots of colorful fruits and vegetables, and even some legumes and gluten-free grains (in small quantities). If you have too much gas, try the FODMAPs protocol for 6 weeks and regroup.

- Eat wild-caught seafood or pasture-raised, grass-fed meats in moderation.

- Implement some kind of stress management regimen like meditation or exercise.

- After 2 months, if you're feeling great, reintroduce some triggers one at a time using the food diary method in Chapter 9.

- Cut out processed foods forever; they're garbage.

Toxic Trigger Foods to Eliminate

It's very hard to look at foods you've had a relationship with and say good-bye. But if you want to achieve optimal gut health, you *must* say good-bye. Think of a relationship with a needy person who drains you of all your energy, wakes you up in the middle of the night with drama and complaints, and gives you nothing in return but a couple of cheap laughs at someone else's expense. Do you really want to hang out with that person? We hope you don't. Life's too short for that kind of nonsense. If food is toxic to your gut and your brain, then ditch it like the dead weight it is.

We know we were a little rough back there about toxic food, but tough love is needed every now and then. The good news is you might not have to give up these foods forever because they might not turn out to be triggers for you after all. Or, it may turn out that once your intestinal hyper-permeability calms down, your system will be able to tolerate these foods again. But you won't know any of that until you quit them for a while. Several weeks at least. To go back to our relationship metaphors from before, tell your possible trigger foods that you, "need some space."

Casein and Lactose

Casein and lactose are the proteins and sugars in milk. After a few weeks, you can try ghee, butter, and fermented dairy that is very low in these two substances. But for several weeks give your body a break. Remember the discussion of casomorphins back in Chapter 7? Milk proteins aren't digested properly if your enterocytes are sickly, and your gut is leaky. Instead, you send those opiate-like substances to your brain. You might literally be addicted to milk protein. Kick the habit and see how you feel.

Try not to get sucked into the "healthy junk food trap." Even processed foods that boast dairy-free claims can still contain other triggers, namely sugar. There are also many dairy-free products that still sneak casein in there. If you feel like you need a "milk-like-fix," stick to whole-food, highly nutritious replacements for dairy like unsweetened almond, cashew, coconut, and hemp milks.

Gluten

Gluten can produce the same kind of opiate-like substances that casein does. Additionally, gluten releases that magical zonulin that is the gatekeeper for the tight junctions that help maintain proper permeability for your intestinal lining. Don't send it into overdrive while you're trying to heal your gut. Ditch the gluten and then try it several weeks down the road to test it as one of your personal triggers. Even if it turns out you can tolerate gluten, it's good to give your body a break from all that zonulin and make sure you're sealing your gut properly.

With all the recent gluten-free diet crazes there is a smorgasbord of gluten-free products in nearly every supermarket. It's all too easy to look at the selection and feel tempted to indulge. After all, it's gluten free, right? The unfortunate truth about many of those products is that the processed gluten product is simply swapped out for another processed carbohydrate that is gluten free. Some of these common ingredients include rice flours, sugar, potato starch, soy, buckwheat, and tapioca flours. Some of these ingredients may negatively affect the gut microbiota just as much as gluten.

> **GUT WISE**
>
> Another indicator that you might have a gluten problem is a nasty skin condition called dermatitis herpetiformis. It looks like a bad case of hives or poison ivy and is just as irritating and itchy. Because it looks like so many other skin conditions, it's often misdiagnosed. If you've been having digestive issues and you have some skin eruptions, you may have undiagnosed gluten enteropathy. Get tested by your doctor.

We're not saying to never eat gluten-free bread or cookies; just do so very sparingly. Even better, to satisfy those inevitable cravings learn how to make your own wholesome baked goods and have complete quality control.

Refined Sugars and Carbs, Trans Fats, and Table Salt

Basically everything containing refined sugars, refined carbs, trans fats, or table salts is considered a processed food. Any one of these by themselves is bad for you, but so many processed foods contain all of them. If you eat something out of a bag or a box, check the ingredients very carefully. Even if it says "all natural," they sneak stuff in there that is far from wholesome. Nasty salts are hidden in ingredients like "yeast extract" and "hydrolyzed soy protein."

> **YOU ARE WHAT YOU EAT**
>
> Monosodium glutamate (MSG) is a dubious food additive. It manipulates one of our taste buds' favorite senses called *umami*. Your taste buds detect sweet, sour, salty, bitter, and umami, which detects glutamates in food. Glutamate is an essential amino acid your body needs. MSG mimics that natural substance, but it's a little "off" like trans fats are off. Your taste buds are programmed to register what you're eating as nutritious, but MSG is far from it. MSG stimulates insulin production and produces substances in the body that affect the brain in the same way Valium does. MSG is addictive and unhealthy.

White sugars, pastas, rice, and breads are all toxic to the body and need to be tossed. They feed pathogenic bacteria and have high glycemic loads that contribute to candida overgrowth (not to mention diabetes and heart disease).

Eat Well to Restore Your Body

Whenever we undertake a health plan, we often focus too much on what we can't do and what we can't have. While it's true there are many things you shouldn't eat, most of them are man-made concoctions that are better described as "foodlike substances" rather than actual food. Let's accentuate the positive by discussing all the yummy things you *can* eat that will soothe the gut and contribute to overall health.

Fruits, Vegetables, Grains, and Proteins

After you trash the toxic triggers, you're free to try what remains, which are fresh, whole foods. Eat lots of vegetables and some ripe fruits. Fruits do contain sugars, and this can promote some bacteria growth and even SIBO, so don't eat too much of it. Balance out your food groups. A basic place to start when building your meals is to take a standard dinner plate and divide it in three. Proteins, nonstarchy carbs, and starchy carbs should occupy equal portions of this plate. An example of this would be a plate filled with one third sweet potatoes, one third salmon, one third kale and melon slices.

Portion division will give you an idea of how not to overload on any one type of food and feed your gut the diversity of whole foods it really craves for optimal health and balance. If you do this, you won't have to necessarily cut out large swaths of food from your diet, unless you find you have a reaction. Keep that food diary, and you'll know for sure. A food diary will also help you track if there are some higher FODMAPs foods that you need to go easy on.

Make sure you get protein from a variety of responsibly raised sources. Try lean meats, nuts, legumes, and eggs, and exercise the portion control that makes them the complement to the meal rather than the main event. If you exercise a lot, you may find you need more protein and carbs, and you may have to adjust your ratios and portions to find the individual results that make you feel your best. Larger portions of gluten-free grains like brown rice and quinoa, healthy fats like coconut and avocado, more lean meat, and extra mineral-rich sea salts B_{12} might be necessary if you're an athlete or have strenuous workouts.

 YOU ARE WHAT YOU EAT

A note about eggs: these poor guys get a bad reputation as elevators of cholesterol levels, but the cholesterol in eggs helps your body build cell membranes and repair immune cells after they fight infection. The amino acids and vitamin B_{12} in eggs are beneficial and easily absorbed by the body. The real bad cholesterol culprit is processed food. So enjoy your eggs for breakfast, lunch, or dinner.

Learn to read your metabolism by tracking your energy levels, along with other symptoms, as you keep a food diary. Your goal is to be free of negative symptoms and feel full of energy. You may find you need a few more carbs or a larger portion of protein in order to feel your best. Customizing your healthy gut plan is about trial and error just as much as it is about following guidelines to give you a yardstick by which to measure your choices. Adjust your portions so that you're not starved between meals and not stuffed immediately afterward. Read over the symptoms of healthy digestion in Chapter 2 and make sure that you are on track.

The Importance of Fermented Foods

Fermented foods have been used worldwide as a part of a well-rounded diet. They help with digestion and normalize our gut microbiome by replenishing the good bacteria populations. Fermented foods are a daily dose of bacterial reinforcement troops that keep pathogenic bacteria, and even parasites, in check. And while probiotic supplements can be effective, most of them aren't close to the effectiveness of good old-fashioned food. This is probably because the bacteria in foods have a better chance to survive the stomach acid than the ones in capsules.

Sauerkraut, olives, kefir, matzoon, lassi, gioddu, yogurt, cheese, miso, natto, tempeh, kumiss, and kimchi are all fermented foods are rich in naturally occurring probiotics that promote gut health. There are so many more, but this list will get you started. Make sure to opt for organic versions of these foods. You can even ferment some of them yourself. You might find the word *cultured* used interchangeably with *fermented,* especially when dealing with dairy. *Cultured* simply means you add a mix of bacteria "starter," and fermented foods are made when you depend on the bacteria already in the food to multiply and do the fermentation work.

Adding fermented foods to your diet should be done gradually to avoid uncomfortable bloating, and also to avoid some other detox symptoms that can arise when too many of the bad guys living in your gut die off at one time (more on this in Chapter 16). You can start with just 1 teaspoon of these foods at each meal and then work up to larger portions that you can tolerate without any negative digestive symptoms. The goal is to feed your good microbes so your microbes help heal your gut.

The History and Power of Bone Broths

So what is bone broth anyway? A broth is made with some meat simmering in water for a few hours. Stock is made when you add the actual bones with the meat and water and simmer for even longer. A bone broth is produced when you simmer bones with a little meat on them in water for around 24 hours. The end result is a concoction chock-full of nutrients and amino acids that are easily absorbed by the body.

Bone broths are a staple in nearly every cuisine worldwide with traditions stretching back thousands of years. Why are they so pervasive? They're good for you, and they're cheap! They're such an easy way to utilize every part of an animal and drag those nutrients out of even the toughest parts. When you take a day (or 2 or 3) to cook down tough meat, tendons, ligaments, bones, marrow, knuckles, skin, and feet (yes, feet), all the good stuff comes out. In fact, some of the compounds in old-fashioned bone broth are what some supplement companies charge quite a pretty penny for. You could make your own superfood at home for so much less. (We show you how in Chapter 14.)

So what is that magical stuff in bone broth, and why is it so good for you?

- **Proline and collagen:** Promote healthy skin, bones, tendons, and the tissues that protect our organs

- **Gelatin:** Helps soothe and even repair the gut lining

- **Glycine and sulfur compounds:** Aid in detoxing, nutrient absorption, help methylation, have anti-inflammatory effects, and aid glutathione production

- **Magnesium:** Helps calcium absorption

- **Calcium:** Bone, muscle, cell, and cardiac health and function

- **Glucosamine and chondroitin:** Contribute to joint maintenance and health

There are so many nutrients on that list that are marketed as high-end supplements. You could pay a lot of money for them, and they still wouldn't be as easily absorbed by the body as they will be in a bone broth. Chicken bone broth exclusively contains another amino acid to add to this list: cysteine. Cysteine is a powerful antioxidant that boosts the immune system and helps glutathione levels. Yes, Grandma was certainly right about chicken soup.

ASK THE EXPERTS

Good broth will resurrect the dead.

—South American proverb

Customizing to Your Dietary Needs

Although some foundational bacteria and digestive processes are universal, the exact combination of bacteria in the gut and the portions of fermented, FODMAPs, or trigger foods *you* can handle are unique to you. Figuring out what works best for the conditions of your body with your personal medical history and environment is like cracking your healthy gut code.

Using the food diary method we suggested in Chapter 9, get rid of the most common trigger foods first, then figure out your *personal* triggers by reintroducing the foods back into your diet—one at a time for one week at a time. After you've reintroduced everything you wanted to try, you might find there are some foods you can only tolerate in small amounts or not at all.

You don't want to start all over again with reinjuring the gut lining and launching into leaky gut, SIBO, food sensitivities, discomfort, or inflammation. But you also don't want to feel so deprived of your favorite foods that you end up bingeing on them and causing further damage. One of the best things you can do if you have trigger foods is find replacements for them.

Find healthy alternatives, and if you don't like them keep trying small tastes of them over time. You might find you love the whole-food substitutes for your triggers. Dairy is usually the hardest for people to give up. But if cow's milk is your trigger, try almond or hemp milk. If you miss cream-based sauces, try recipes that substitute with cashew butter; it really gives a wonderful texture that will remind you of your old favorites. If you're missing ice cream, chop up a few bananas and throw them in the freezer for several hours. Place the frozen banana chunks in a food processor with a little vanilla extract and cinnamon for a few minutes, and you have a soft-serve banana treat.

 YOU ARE WHAT YOU EAT

Almond milk has been used in Europe and the Middle East for centuries. In Medieval Europe, it was often used during Lent when dairy was forbidden. And it was regularly use as well since it doesn't go bad as quickly as the milk from cows, goats, or sheep. Almond milk is easy to store and has a long shelf life. It's high in protein and vitamin E and has no lactose. Virtually any recipe you would ordinarily make with cow's milk can be made with almond milk. Like a lot of seemingly "newfangled" health food fads, almond milk actually has a long and glorious history as a nutritious staple.

If you're stubborn about giving up your triggers or reluctant to try something that seems too exotic, you kind of have to approach it like giving a kid vegetables he doesn't want at first. You may have to try small doses of healthy, nutrient-rich foods over and over to acquire the taste for them. And try hard not to buy the processed alternatives whose additives and denatured approach to food will make the substitute almost as bad for you as the trigger.

Essential Herbs and Supplements

If you have intestinal hyperpermeability or other digestive issues, chances are you have trouble absorbing all of the vitamins, minerals, and fatty acids you need. You may have to supplement your diet as your gut lining heals. After around 6 months, you should be able to wean yourself off of powder and pill supplements to your diet. Ideally, all of your nutritional needs should be met with real food, but that isn't always possible if you suffer from chronic digestive issues.

In the short term, taking supplements can help your body heal. Over time, your conditions will become easier to manage, and your intestine can get back on track. Once you feel energized and in control of your gut health, you can wean yourself off of extra supplements if you like, or at least decrease your doses. Depending on your gut microbiota, you may always have to take at least low-level doses of some supplements, but the health benefits are worth the trouble of finding the right combination and doses for you. An integrative practitioner or dietitian can personalize a supplement regimen for you based on your health history. Here's an overview of some of the most important supplements to consider for optimal gut health.

Fatty Acids

There's a lot of talk in health circles these days about omega fatty acids and their importance. They are crucial to your health, and they're not all created equally, nor are they interchangeable. Your body's cells specifically need omega-3 and omega-6 fatty acids, but your body doesn't make them on its own.

One of the biggest problems in the typical modern diet is the intake of too many omega-6 fatty acids from cooking with vegetable oils like canola, corn, and soybean or consuming processed food products containing those oils. These sources contribute to cardiovascular disease and inflammation. The structure of vegetable oils is pretty fragile. The initial process of creating the oils and the heat from cooking damages the fatty acids, and they in turn damage our bodies. We still need omega-6 acids, but in more equal ratios and from healthier sources than what most people consume. Healthier sources of omega-6 are in grass-fed, pasture-raised, and free-range animals.

Typical Westerners consume around 20 times more omega-6s than omega-3s when for optimal health that ratio should be closer to 2:1 or 1:1. What we really need to consume more of, and may need to take supplements of, are omega-3 fatty acids. Fish oil, cod liver oil, and krill oil supplements are excellent sources of omega-3s. We need omega-3s for eye and brain health especially. Gut lining problems compound the problem of absorption, so if you suffer from leaky gut taking an omega-3 supplement is particularly helpful.

Digestive Enzymes

If you have imbalanced gut microbiota, chances are you also have low stomach acid. When you don't have enough stomach acid, pathogenic bacteria can grow on the lining of your stomach the same way they do in the intestine. These microbes then proliferate and digest carbs in the stomach, when that usually wouldn't happen. The fermentation of carbs in your stomach causes uncomfortable gas and harmful acid reflux.

Talk to you integrative practitioner or dietitian about adding HCL with pepsin to your supplement regimen, as these acids can help you stop the carbs from fermenting in your stomach and help it restore the natural pH balance. Other digestive enzymes that can help achieve gut health are amylase, lactase, cellulose, peptidases, proteases, and lipases. These enzymes are all contributed to digestion by the pancreas, but in people with low stomach acid and other digestive issues, the stomach might not be triggering the pancreas to send enough juice. You can buy these enzymes in capsule form. The most effective are those formulas that say "blended" and those from companies who specialize only in digestive enzymes.

Vitamins and Minerals You Need

A compromised gut lining has a harder time absorbing vitamins and minerals. Vitamin A is a big problem in this department. Vitamin A helps with enterocyte regeneration and white blood cell production. Cod liver oil is a good vitamin A supplement, which will cover you for your omega-3s as well as vitamin D. You really should take vitamin A and D together as they don't work properly when the other isn't present; they're kind of codependent that way. If you have too little of one, it creates a surplus of the other that can even be toxic. They balance one another out, and cod liver oil natural supplies you with a correct balance.

GUT WISE

We often down vitamins only when we're sick with the hope they'll rescue our immune systems in large doses at the last minute. At the first sign of a cold there are some things you can do to help you fight it off. Vitamin D and zinc can boost your immune system. Black elderberries have natural anti-viral properties and can be added to juices fresh or can be taken as an extract supplement available at health food stores.

As far as taking multivitamins and lots of extra individual vitamins, the scientific literature leans toward gleaning your vitamins and minerals from food sources. The main reason for this consensus is poor absorption. If you're anemic, you may be prescribed a course of iron, but if your body doesn't have the B_{12} to help it absorb the iron, and if your enterocytes are damaged, then most of your supplement is literally going down the drain. A great way to boost your intake of phytonutrients, antioxidants, vitamins, and minerals is with regular juicing of fresh fruits and veggies. (Look back to Chapter 9 for some specific detox juices for use in the short term that can jump-start your healthy gut diet.)

You can take vitamin supplements, however, if you feel they help boost your energy levels. Certainly some absorption is better than none at all when you're trying to build your body's immune system and get your GI tract in order. When picking out vitamin and mineral supplements, try to find products that contain fulvic acid, as this substance helps improve absorption rates. While you're working toward healing the gut, the most important supplements to take are digestive enzymes and stomach acid support, omega-3s, vitamins D and A, the glutathione support discussed in Chapter 9, and probiotics.

The Power of Probiotics

Cultures the world over have used fermented foods as a healthy contribution to their diets for millennia. You can ferment milk, vegetables, fruit, beans, and even meats and grains. This process makes food easier to preserve and to digest. The process also fosters the growth of bacteria that promote gut health.

Science has been able to isolate many strains of beneficial bacteria produced in these health-promoting foods and offer them as dietary supplements. These strains of bacteria are useful in building a robust and diverse population of gut bacteria that can combat disease and support healthy digestion.

Good Bacteria and Microbiota

There are three main groups of good bacteria you want to ingest to bring balance to your microbiota: lactobacilli, bifidobacteria, and Bacillus subtilis.

Lactobacilli strains produce lactic acid, which lowers the pH of the mucous membranes they inhabit. Lower pH levels make it harder for pathogenic strains to thrive. Lactobacilli also supports immune system functions such as antibody production. These bacteria also help with enterocyte regeneration, which keeps the gut lining healthy.

> **GUT WISE**
>
> It can be hard to find a probiotic that has all three of the major groups you want to ingest. Syntol AMD, manufactured by Arthur Andrew Medical, has eight strains of bacteria in one capsule from all three of the good families you need. To see a comprehensive listing of major commercially available probiotics, and the strains they each contain, visit thecandidadiet.com/list-of-probiotics.

Bifidobacteria are plentiful in the gut (or should be), and they ensure gut health in numerous ways. They produce substances that act like your own personal internal sanitizers to suppress the overgrowth of pathogens. Bifidobacteria also help maintain immunity and the health and integrity of the gut lining. These probiotics are also involved in the production of amino acids and B vitamins and help our intestinal wall absorb iron and vitamin D.

Bacillus subtilis are naturally found in soil. They have proven themselves effective in helping alleviate allergies and autoimmune symptoms. This is largely because of the immune system support they offer. Bacillus subtilis make digestive enzymes and more of those internal sanitizers. This family of bacteria differs from bifidobacteria and lactobacilli in that it isn't a permanent resident of our gut. It's called a transitional microbe. These types of microbes are ingested and hitch a ride to our GI tract via the water we drink and food we eat. But while they're our gut guests, they do great work. They break down material that might be rotting in the gut while keeping pathogens who feed on the same stuff from getting out of control.

Choose the Right Probiotic Supplement

Diverse cultures of probiotics are available in pill and powder form, but you can also get just as many, if not more, probiotics from eating fermented foods. Eating probiotic foods might be difficult for you, however, because they induce a lot of gas. Or you simply might not like their tastes or textures. Often fermented foods beyond yogurt aren't readily available in grocery stores near you, and pill and powder forms may be more convenient. Quality probiotic supplements are available at health food stores, but also from trusted vendors online, so everyone can have access to these microscopic gut-health powerhouses.

Choose a probiotic supplement with a combination of at least the three main groups of probiotic bacteria best for the gut: lactobacilli, bifidobacteria, and Bacillus subtilis. Certainly the supplement you pick can have a lot more variety than these, in fact, the more varied the better. We have hundreds of species in our guts; the more diversified probiotic you find, the better it will be for your gut. You also want to ensure that the formula you choose is concentrated. Read the label to find out how many live bacterial cells are in each gram. You should aim for at least 8 billion per gram. Also research the brand you choose, and make sure they test and guarantee each batch.

Follow the directions for dosing on the packaging and work with a dietitian if you have specific questions about how you should incorporate the probiotics into your routine to maximize their health benefits. A general guideline for adults is to take around 15 billion probiotic cells a day for the first several months of your healthy gut diet. After that, you can decrease to around 8 billion a day. Everyone has a different tolerance level, however, so keep track of how you feel (in your food diary) and reach out to health practitioners for advice.

You also want to decide if you prefer a powder or a pill. If you choose a pill, pick one whose coating isn't too thick or labeled as "enteric." You want your entire GI tract to benefit from the bacteria. The thick coating is designed to withstand stomach acid, but if your gut health is already compromised, you might not be able to break down the coating at all. You'll never get the chance to benefit from those probiotic critters.

The Least You Need to Know

- Start your diet by cutting out gluten, casein, and all refined and processed foods.
- To start, eat equal portions of protein, starchy veggies, and nonstarchy veggies with every meal and then adjust based on how you feel.
- Add foods that soothe and repair the gut lining and its beneficial microbiota, such as fermented foods and bone broths.
- Gradually add former trigger foods and track your progress, find healthy alternatives, and ditch processed foods forever.
- Boost your vitamin intake with freshly pressed juices, cod liver oil, and digestive enzyme supplements.
- Eat fermented foods or choose a high-quality probiotic supplement with lactobacilli, bifidobacteria, and Bacillus subtilis.

CHAPTER 12

Getting Ready for a Healthy Gut

In this chapter, we give you specific guidelines for setting yourself up for healthy gut success. You learn how to get your kitchen ready with staples, basic appliances, and culinary tools. In addition, we provide helpful grocery shopping tips.

Then we tackle one of the biggest monsters of all: eliminating toxins from your home. Most of us don't even realize the toxic waste dump that lives in our bathrooms and under our kitchen sinks. Cleaning supplies and personal-care products are often full of nasty chemicals that can sabotage our health. You learn what they are, how they affect your gut health, and find some healthier alternatives that will complement your healthy gut diet.

In This Chapter

- Detoxing your kitchen and stocking it with staples and healthy gut tools
- Budgeting for a healthy gut
- Grocery shopping strategies
- Replacing toxic personal and home cleaning products with healthy alternatives

Preparing Your Kitchen

One of the first things you need to do to prepare your kitchen for a healthy gut is to prepare the cook's attitude. This is especially true if one of the reasons why you haven't made healthy meal choices in the past was because you felt like you didn't have time to cook healthy meals. The truth is, we usually end up figuring out how to make time for the things we enjoy and are important to us.

If you feel cooking is a time suck, try really hard to think about it differently. What are you giving up to cook? Time online? Watching a rerun you've seen a dozen times? Relaxing? The truth is that cooking can be relaxing once you get into the habit of having healthy items and a well-equipped kitchen. Think of all you have to gain in gut health and in family time spent around a table eating more farm-to-table meals prepared with care. Think of the longer and healthier life you'll live free from disease.

Preparing your kitchen and your home for a healthy gut is essential to the success of a healthy gut regimen. Eliminating temptation and having healthy foods and a stock of recipes and staples on hand will set you up to succeed in your healthy gut plan.

Let Go of Triggers

Purging your kitchen of unhealthy foods will eliminate temptation later. If you don't do this, you will have the constant dilemma of knowing those foods are ready to eat—taxing your will power. This means getting out a large garbage bag and chucking processed foods, sugary snacks, unhealthy cooking oils, nonfat commercial dairy, white breads, white rice, white pastas, white sugar, and refined table salt. We know this is counterintuitive. Most of us grew up in households where wasting foods is sinful. This is not the same as wasting food. This is literally taking out the trash. What you are throwing away really isn't food but foodlike substances detrimental to your health.

If your family is not supportive in this kind of drastic measure, take heart and be strong. You can still be successful. Instead of chucking everything, try to make separate areas in your kitchen where you keep your healthy options so you get used to going to your spot. This is a kind of "out of sight, out of mind" tactic. If you are the main meal-preparer in the family, try not to get sucked into making separate unhealthy meals for them and then a healthy option for yourself. This will cause temptation for you. Simply prepare healthy meals and invite everyone to partake or fend for themselves.

Who knows? You may provide the inspiration for other family members to join you as they'll probably be curious about your choices. If they're negative, remember that you can control your own health and have a buddy outside the home who can encourage you.

GUT WISE

Remember to build a health professional team for support, as we discussed in Chapter 4. See Appendix B for online support forums as well. You need all the help and support you can get from a variety of sources.

Kitchen Tools

Never underestimate the power of good kitchen knives. This is an investment that will last for years. Chopping vegetables and meats will be a daily task, so you might as well make it easy and pleasurable. Well-made sharp knives make an enormous difference. A high-quality blender also makes sauces, salad dressings, nut spreads, blended soups, and smoothies a breeze to whip up.

You'll need pots and pans of various sizes for steaming and sautéing. Some 4- to 6-quart pots are good for everyday use, but be sure at least one is a 16-quart stockpot for making bone broths and for batch cooking. A stockpot often has a steamer, which is slightly smaller pot (with holes) that fits snugly inside the larger stockpot. A nice pasta pot is often outfitted with a steamer and can be used for making stock. When you're making bone broths or vegetable broth, all you'll need to do when cooking time is done is carefully lift the steamer out of the pot and toss out its contents. You may have to strain the broth through a cheesecloth if there are still particles leftover, afterward you can enjoy the nutrient-dense broth left behind.

No matter which brand of pots and pans you choose, do not use nonstick pans. They're made with harmful substances known to leach into food. Stainless-steel cookware works best.

Slow cookers are great for stews and soups and even bone broths. These nourishing staples will become some of your go-to meals. Broths also serve as the basis for sauces or a cooking medium for veggies and meats. You can use slow cookers while you're at work or when you don't have time to worry about watching a stockpot. When you cook vegetables in water or broths, most of their nutrients remain in the soup. Slow cookers can hold large enough batches to have leftovers, which can save you time during the work week.

Pressure cookers are another time saver. One major benefit to these devices is that they actually help vegetables retain more nutrients than steaming in steel colanders over boiling water. The big win with pressure cookers is shortened cooking time. They look like big stockpots with locks on them. They work by using steam pressure to increase the boiling point of water, which cooks food faster and forces moisture into food at a quicker pace. Pressure cookers range in price from small models that go for around $60 to larger mammoths the size of microwaves that can cost a couple hundred bucks. Including this piece of equipment is at the discretion of your counter or cabinet space and your budget.

Juicers are also wonderful to have on hand, but they can be expensive and bulky. However, the nutrients derived from freshly juiced fruits and vegetables are great for detoxing and daily gut health. If you find you get bloated easily, juicing can be a great option for you to get the nutrients from fresh produce. When you juice fruits and vegetables, you don't get any of the fiber, which although essential to gut health can cause bloating and feed some bad gut bacteria. Like the pressure cooker, this piece of equipment is at your discretion.

Store homemade stocks and yogurts in glass storage containers to make the most of leftovers. There are no plastics to leech into food, and the bottom line is that food stored in glass tastes better and keeps longer than plastic storage systems ever did.

Essential Staples

Weekly food shopping and meal planning should include a variety of in-season produce, fresh proteins, and healthy carbs. There are also staples that you should always have in your kitchen Staples complement your fresh ingredients, add flavor to them healthfully, thicken sauces, add zest to salad dressings, and provide some go-to standbys to accompany your meals.

One way to be sure you're always well stocked with staples is to take note of when you're low and immediately add those items to a running grocery list you keep somewhere visible in your kitchen, like on your pantry or refrigerator door.

Here's a list of staple items you should always have on hand:

In your pantry, keep the following: almond butter, almond flour, almond milk, apple cider vinegar, baking soda, balsamic vinegar, fresh bananas, whole-grain brown rice, organic chicken and vegetable broths (homemade is best, but if you run out it's good to have some in a pinch), cashews, coconut flour, coconut milk, unrefined extra virgin coconut oil, cold-pressed extra virgin olive oil, garlic, ghee, a large variety of spices, raw honey, onions, quinoa, Celtic or Himalayan sea salt, shallots, tahini (sesame seed paste), canned or packaged wild-caught seafood without additives (tuna, salmon, crab, and clams), organic vanilla extract, and dried beans.

In your refrigerator, keep the following: in-season fruits and veggies, Bragg's amino acids, organic egg whites, lemon and lime juices, organic salad dressings made with cold-pressed olive oils, fresh greens, organic free-range eggs, and homemade or organic full-fat yogurt.

In your freezer, keep the following: peeled and chopped bananas (for cooking and smoothies), berries, bone broths, leftovers (soups and sauces freeze well), organic free-ranging meats (such as whole chicken and chicken breasts), wild-caught fish, and various veggies without additives.

YOU ARE WHAT YOU EAT

If lettuce and greens are starting to go bad, put two handfuls in a freezer storage bag and freeze them for quick and easy smoothies as a breakfast or snack. The greens actually freeze very nicely!

Keeping stocked with these staples will help you create gut-friendly meals even when you're cooking on the fly. Keep these in mind when you're building your meal plans and grocery lists. Even if you're pressed for time, you can always sauté veggies and protein and throw them over brown rice or make some fresh tuna salad over a bed of lettuce and a quick bowl of quinoa flavored with leftover bone broth.

Grocery Shopping Strategies

You need to make a realistic schedule for when you're going to go grocery shopping. Think about your obligations for a regular week and plan on the best day and time that will work for you. The last thing you want is to be so pressed for time that you run into the store looking for quick and easy options, which could land you in the dangerous realm of processed meals in the freezer section. Don't just head to the store with wishful thinking and good intentions in your pocket. You need a plan.

The best place to start is to map out your meals for the week. Build your meal ideas around fresh seasonal veggies and fruits and proteins. Remember the dinner plate divided into three parts. Think, "What will I have for my starchy veggie, nonstarchy veggie, protein, and maybe some fruit on the side or for dessert?" Take into consideration how many people you're cooking for and how many work and school lunches you may have to prepare.

You can always make extra-large dinners, so you're guaranteed leftovers for lunches (that's where stocks, soups, and good thermoses can come in handy). Some weeks you might have more time than others. During weeks when you find you have more time, consider cooking large batches of soaps, stews, and roasted poultry, so you can freeze them for the busier weeks that are bound to come. (We'll have more on batch cooking in Part 4.)

If what you're hankering for isn't in season, you can plan on grabbing those ingredients from the frozen section. Stay away from too many canned goods as they are usually high in sodium and preservatives. After you have your meal plans for the week, you can build a grocery list based on the ingredients you'll need that aren't already in your pantry or refrigerator. Always go grocery shopping with a list, and always eat something before you go. The last thing you need is a rumbling stomach and aisle after aisle of temptations to fight.

Make a Budget

You want to be realistic, but you also want to be healthy. When deciding on your food budget, you need to also consider the costs of not eating healthy, which are inevitably more doctor visits and medical costs. While those consequences might be in the more distant future, when it comes to your health you want to play the long game. If you need immediacy to appreciate benefits, think of the mental and monetary costs of missing work because you're immune system and gut aren't functioning properly. Priorities are everything in life.

The first step you should do to make an effective monthly grocery budget is figure out what you're already spending on food. The easiest way to do this is by simply saving all your food-related receipts for a month and then tallying them up. That means not just your grocery bill, but any and all food purchases you've made including convenience store snacks, coffee shop drinks, work lunches, and all restaurant and bar bills. Once you know what you spend each month, you'll have a number for managing what you can afford.

GUT WISE

According to a 2012 survey in the *Christian Science Monitor*, the average American spends $232 on 18.2 restaurant meals a month. Cutting down on eating out can free up more money for healthier foods you can prepare and control yourself.

After you've set that monthly dollar amount, there are some guidelines you can follow to spend that money wisely. Although you may find some grocery-store items that you can cut from your budget, there could be other items that are always worth the added expense because of their health benefits.

Here are some grocery budget guidelines:

- Food items that are a must and shouldn't be skimped on include fresh produce, responsibly raised free-range meats, gluten-free whole grains, full-fat organic yogurt with live cultures, unrefined extra virgin coconut and olive oils, and raw honey.

- Plan your meals, make a weekly list based on that plan. (We discuss more on meal planning in Chapter 13.)

- Eat out less often. Restaurants are more fun when they're the exception not the rule.

- Keep a running list of what you run out of in your refrigerator and pantry to avoid under- or overshopping.

- Avoid the coupon and sale traps that tempt you to trade your best-laid meal plans for a deal. If it's not on your grocery list, you don't need it.

- If it's on your list and it's on sale, count your blessings and stock up if you have the space and it's a nonperishable item that you know you'll use before it expires.

Shop the Perimeter

You should spend most of your time at the grocery store in the produce section, health food section (usually in supermarket chains), and the frozen food aisle. The center aisles are full of tempting processed junk. Only go down the center aisles for items like vinegar, baking soda, spices, garbage bags, etc.

GUT WISE

Remember those apps we mentioned for keeping a food diary? There are also apps to keep you on track at the grocery store. They can keep your lists, scan barcodes to check if items contain the triggers you deem to be off limits, and more.

If an item comes in a box, bag, or a jar, read the ingredients and nutritional information carefully. The fewer ingredients, the better. If a food is highly processed, it's most likely devoid of nutritional value and not worth your money or time. Some exceptions to this are organic tomato sauces and low-sodium condiments free of refined sugars like corn syrup or refined carbohydrates like wheat flour.

YOU ARE WHAT YOU EAT

Here are some helpful tips on reading labels as you grocery shop. Ingredients are listed in descending order of volume. In other words, the first ingredient makes up the bulk of the product. Steer clear of hydrogenated fats, corn syrups and other sweeteners, and white or wheat flours (whole-wheat flours are okay in moderation if well tolerated). If the number of milligrams (mg) of sodium in a product outnumber the calories in the product, put it back on the shelf.

Choose Local and Organic

Buying local means fresher food. Quite simply, it just doesn't have far to travel. It's also less likely to be full of preservatives and harmful sprays used on produce to survive long trips without spoiling.

YOU ARE WHAT YOU EAT

The average apple on grocery store shelves worldwide is between 9 and 14 months old! They're picked, waxed, and sprayed with a chemical called 1-methylcyclopropene that slows the ripening and oxidation processes. This is why typical grocery store apples can often be mealy. After a few months they lose their natural antioxidant content. Another reason to eat local, in-season produce that is preferably organic.

There are requirements growers and food manufacturers must meet before they can label their food "organic." According to the regulations of the USDA National Organic Program, the term "organic" can only be officially applied to:

> [M]eat, poultry, eggs, and dairy products … from animals that are given no antibiotics or growth hormones. Organic food is produced without using most conventional pesticides; fertilizers made with synthetic ingredients or sewage sludge; bioengineering; or ionizing radiation. Before a product can be labeled "organic," a government-approved certifier inspects the farm where the food is grown to make sure the farmer is following all the rules necessary to meet USDA organic standards. Companies that handle or process organic food before it gets to your local supermarket or restaurant must be certified, too.

So how do you apply this knowledge when buying produce and other food products at the grocery store? There are different labeling categories products can attain from the USDA. If the label says "100% Organic," it's either an organically grown fruit or vegetable or product made with 100 percent organic ingredients. If it simply says "Organic," it's made with 95 to 99 percent organic ingredients. If the label reads "Made with Organic Ingredients," at least 70 percent of its total ingredients must be organic, and the other 30 percent must be natural with no GMOs added. Less than 70 percent of organic products aren't allowed to have the term "organic" listed on the front packaging.

Buying organic can be expensive if all the produce in your cart bears that label. But if your budget allows, go for it. If you're on a tight budget, choose organic fruits and vegetables for those you plan to eat with the peel or skin on. Nonorganic produce can retain toxins from pesticides in their skin no matter how hard you wash them, so be sure to peel those before you eat.

The other line item to allocate your budget dollars to are on high-quality organic proteins such as full-fat dairy, raw nuts, and free-ranging meats. Organic meats will be free of antibiotics and growth hormones. Besides being great for your gut, they'll be fresher and taste better and will make healthy toxin-free bone broths.

Minimizing Home Toxins

Our technologies and the pollutants they've produced have advanced faster than our bodies can evolve to keep up, and that includes our detox systems. So we have to make the effort to detox our home to combat this problem. By decreasing the load we place on our stressed-out liver, we can optimize its ability to filter pathogens and boost our immune system, which will place less stress on our gut while it's healing.

> **GUT WISE**
>
> Surprising things you can do to jump-start your immune system while your gut heals include swimming in the ocean, having a pet, and walking or working outside.

One way you can decrease your exposure to toxins is where you have the most control over them—in your home. Most of the products we use to clean our homes, and ourselves, contain toxic substances. Over time, exposure to these chemicals builds up in our system and overtaxes the liver and other filtering systems in our bodies.

You can be kinder to your body by making more conscientious choices when you buy new flooring, carpeting, or paint for your home. Be mindful of the water, air, and soil quality where you live, work, and spend time. You can also purchase new cleaning products and personal-care products from companies that are conscientious and use natural nontoxic alternatives. Better yet, you can make a lot of your own cleansers and beauty products and have complete quality control.

Indoor Air Quality

In modern societies, we've come to live a largely indoor, sedentary existence. This takes a toll on the mind, body, and spirit. Getting outside reduces allergies over time, increases blood flow, and boosts endorphins released into the blood. Exposure to soil actually improves the composition of the microbiota on our skin and in our bodies.

> **GUT WISE**
>
> You probably already know that plants expel oxygen and absorb carbon dioxide. They also absorb other toxins. Improve the air quality in your home by introducing houseplants wherever you have space. If you're not particularly "green-thumbed," choose low-maintenance varieties like philodendrons or spider plants. You'll breathe easier and improve ambience at the same time.

Our homes are too often sealed off to the outside world with recycled air pumping through vents that might be full of mold and allergens. There are those of us who even have a gene that can cause us to be hyper-reactive to mold, developing respiratory and brain-gut axis problems as a result. Avoid this by keeping the humidity levels in your home between 30 and 50 percent. We want to be energy efficient, but on nice days open the windows and let the sunshine in. Even on the hottest days, you can open some windows for a little while in the morning. This will cut down on mold and let fresh air in.

Reduce Heavy Metal Exposure

Whether it's through the consumption of GMOs, trans fats, contaminated fish, or even the use of common personal-care products, we are exposed to heavy metals that build up in our system. Over time, these metals can disrupt nutrient absorption in the gut lining and can cause problems in the kidneys as well as the nervous and cardiovascular systems.

 YOU ARE WHAT YOU EAT

Juices made with dark leafy greens and tomato and lemon help filter out heavy metals. Carrot, beetroot, and celery juice is a good combination for metal detox and liver health in general.

Staying away from GMOs, trans fats, and compounds like soy protein isolate will definitely cut down on the build-up of aluminum in your system. Cadmium is also another major heavy metal concern because it's found in soils that have been contaminated by mining and industry. It's also found in cigarettes. Cadmium is a gut irritant and a known carcinogen. It makes its way into grains, legumes, and leafy greens. You can minimize your exposure to too much cadmium by only eating organic varieties of these foods and steering clear of cigarette smoke.

Look for Healthier Cleaning Products or Make Your Own

If you have any doubt about the toxicity of your cleaning products, take a look at both the ingredients and the cautionary statements. The warnings on some of these products are downright frightening. You don't have to use poison to clean your home when there are plenty of healthy options out there. You can either spring for cleaners with natural ingredients you recognize by name, or you can make your own. The acids in vinegar and lemon juice kill germs. Safe compounds like alcohol and borax can help you degrease and disinfectant your kitchen and bathroom.

There are plenty of conscientious companies that sell organic and all-natural cleaners with no unpronounceable ingredients. Or you could try one of our recipes for cleaning your home without any harmful toxins.

Window and Glass Cleaner

There is no need for ammonia fumes when you can use these three simple ingredients. (Yield: about 4 cups)

$3^1/_2$ cups water $^1/_4$ cup rubbing alcohol
$^1/_3$ cup white vinegar

1. Combine water, white vinegar, and rubbing alcohol in a large glass jar or clean plastic spray bottle.

2. Shake well before using.

3. You can either dampen a cloth with the solution and apply it to glass surfaces or use the spray bottle the same way you would a store-bought glass cleaner.

Disinfectant

Ditch the bleach and other harsh chemicals with this simple and aromatic cleaner. (Yield: 3 cups)

Lemon, lime, orange, or grapefruit   3 cups white vinegar
    citrus peels (your choice)

1. Place citrus peels and white vinegar in a 1-quart glass jar, and put the lid on it.

2. Keep the mixture in a cabinet; it should dark and cool. Shake the jar once a day for 2 weeks. The mixture will actually ferment a bit.

3. At the end of 2 weeks, run the mixture through a strainer to remove peels and put citrus-infused vinegar back into the jar or a clean spray bottle.

4. To disinfect surfaces, use 1 part cleaner to 3 parts water. You can either dampen a cloth with the solution and apply it to nonporous surfaces like countertops or use a spray bottle the same way you would a store-bought, all-purpose cleaner.

Oven Cleaner

Oven cleaners are some of the most toxic home-cleaning products on the market. Why not make this one instead, that's so safe you could drink it. (Yield: around $1\frac{1}{2}$ cups)

$\frac{1}{2}$ cup baking soda $\frac{1}{2}$ to $\frac{3}{4}$ cup white vinegar
3 to $3\frac{1}{2}$ TB. water

1. In a bowl, combine baking soda and 1 tablespoon water. Add more water, a little at a time, until you have a thick paste almost the consistency of frosting.

2. Remove your oven racks and "frost" your oven's interior surfaces, especially where it's really stained or greasy. A flat plastic spatula works well for this. Avoid getting any cleaner on the heating elements. Let the mixture sit in the oven for 8 to 12 hours or overnight.

3. Use damp paper towels to wipe off the paste.

4. Dampen some paper towels with white vinegar, or put the vinegar in a spray bottle and lightly spray the inside the oven. This may create some white foam in the areas where you still have baking soda remnants, which is fine. The foaming action will break down the remaining gunk.

5. Continue to wipe down the surfaces until all baking soda and vinegar residue are gone.

Garbage Disposal Cleaner

Garbage disposals are fantastic, but over time tiny bits of food and grease can build up on the elements and in your pipes. This can lead to functional problems with the disposal, and it can also lead to unpleasant odors. Clean your disposal with this quick cleaner once every 2 weeks to once a month, and it and your pipes will stay in great shape. (Yield: 1 use)

$\frac{1}{2}$ cup baking soda $\frac{1}{2}$ cup lemon juice or $\frac{1}{2}$ small lemon
1 cup white vinegar

1. Pour baking soda down the drain.

2. Slowly pour white vinegar down the drain, and let foam sit for at least 10 minutes.

3. Finish by pouring in the lemon juice or dropping half a small lemon into the disposal and running water as you run the disposal. This naturally disinfects and deodorize your disposal.

Borax Recipes

Our grandmothers and great grandmothers used borax on a regular basis. With the onset of commercial cleaners, it's gone out of fashion even though it's much safer and more environmentally friendly than the toxic cleaners that consist of harsh chemicals. You shouldn't eat the stuff—in fact, we show you how you can use it as a natural pesticide. But it's certainly safe to use to clean your toilet, carpet, laundry, and more. Here are some basic borax recipes and uses Grandma would approve of:

> **Toilet Cleaner:** Measure 1 cup borax and pour into your toilet. Let it sit for 8 hours (or overnight). Scrub the toilet clean with a toilet brush.

> **Tub Cleanser:** Sprinkle it onto a brush or sponge, and scrub the tub the same way you would with a commercial tub cleanser. Rinse clean with water.

> **Mold and Milder Remover:** Mix equal parts borax and water and spackle it onto the moldy areas. Let it sit for 8 to 12 hours. Wipe off with paper towels, and rinse clean with water.

GUT WISE

Borax is the common name for sodium tetraborate, a substance left behind when seasonal lakes evaporate year after year.

Clean Up Your Personal Products

Personal products come into direct contact with our skin. Recent science demonstrates that toxins are absorbed through the skin, sometimes even more thoroughly than through the digestive system. What we put on our skin can travel directly to the bloodstream, bypassing the liver and its detoxifying powers. This is especially troubling because the cosmetics and toiletry industries are not as tightly regulated as food.

As awareness about toxicity rises, this might change (especially with such actions as The Personal Care Products Safety Act introduced in the U.S. Congress in 2013 and 2015). In the meantime, we need to examine our exposure and the risks involved with these products.

The average Western man uses 9 toiletry products a day, while most women use between 12 and 15. Using conventional commercially produced personal-care products exposes you to thousands of chemicals. This exposure has cumulative effects. In the span of 1 year, you can absorb up to 5 pounds of toxins through your skin just from your personal products. We need to educate ourselves about the products we decide to apply to our skin.

Some of the toxins in beauty products are dangerous, even carcinogenic. For example, there are large numbers of breast cancer cases involving the outer quadrants of the breast. This quadrant is near lymph nodes routinely exposed to the aluminum chloride in most commercially produced antiperspirants. Women who shave their armpits and apply deodorants containing aluminum compounds unwittingly introduce a toxin to their bodies while simultaneously suppressing their bodies' abilities to sweat the toxin out. It just gets stored there in your lymphatic system until it gets into the bloodstream to wreak havoc on your estrogen levels and mutate cells on a genetic level.

Deodorant

Ditch the toxic aluminum levels in commercially produced antiperspirants, and make this instead. To apply this natural deodorant, use your fingers to spread a thin layer on your underarm area as if it were a moisturizer. It should not stain your clothing, but check an inconspicuous area on easily stained fabrics such as silk. (Yield: about $3/4$ cup)

3 TB. arrowroot

3 TB. baking soda

6 TB. coconut oil

A few drops of essential oils: lavender, vanilla, lemongrass, ylang ylang, frankincense, cedarwood, lemon, rosemary, or sandalwood (optional)

1. In a small bowl, combine arrowroot and baking soda.

2. Mash coconut oil into mixture using a fork.

3. Add essential oils (if desired), and stir to combine.

4. Store in a lidded glass container at room temperature in your bathroom cabinet for up to 1 year.

GUT WISE

Reading labels is every bit as important for personal-care products as it is for the food you eat. Some of the substances allowed even in baby wash and shampoos are known irritants and toxins. You have to take it upon yourself to be an informed consumer.

Here are some of the most common toxic substances included in personal-care products and their known and suspected side effects:

Butylated hydroxyanisole/hydroxytoluen: These substances are common ingredients in lotions and cosmetics. They've been linked to kidney, thyroid and liver issues, and are suspected carcinogens.

Diethanolamine: This foaming substance is often present in soaps, shampoos, and lotions. It's a known skin and eye irritant, but more importantly is a suspected carcinogen.

Fragrance and parfum: Labels are actually allowed to simply list this word to signify any number of additives that enhance the smell of a lotion, cosmetics, perfume, shampoo, conditioner, face mask, etc. These substances can be anything from chemicals in the phthalate family to neurotoxins. They can induce allergic reactions and immune system problems.

Imidazolidinyl urea: This is a known irritant and allergen. It stays on the skin for hours even after being rinsed off with water, increasing its opportunity to be absorbed by your skin cells. This is quite troubling as it releases formaldehyde, a known carcinogen. It's a common ingredient in hair dye, shaving cream, face masks, deodorant, and cosmetics.

Parabens: These microbial preservers are in so many products and have been linked to cancer and interruptions in normal hormone function. These are very common in cosmetics; hair-care products; and face, body, and shaving lotions. The good news is that many personal-care products now proudly boast a "paraben-free" label, but check the rest of the contents for other offenders from this list.

Petrolatum: This is petroleum jelly—a product that people have used for over 100 years. The issue is more about how the substance is frequently contaminated with polycyclic aromatic hydrocarbons (PAHs), which are known carcinogens and allergens. Petrolatum is in many hair- and lip-care products.

Phthalates (diethyl phthalate, dibutyl phthalate, dimethyl phthalate): These compounds are also used to make plastics and vinyl. They interrupt normal hormone function and production. They're a common ingredient in cosmetics and also found in toys, toothbrushes, and insecticides. Whether or not they cause cancer hasn't been established, but the substance did cause liver tumors in mice when the substance was applied to their skin in small amounts every day for 2 years. Phthalate exposure in general can cause respiratory and GI tract problems and even spur an early onset of puberty.

Polyethylene glycols (PEGs): These petroleum-based compounds have impurities that have affected kidney and liver function in animal studies. They're often added to lotions and shampoos.

p-Phenylenediamine: This is a common coal tar dye found in hair dye and lipstick. Sometimes it's listed instead as color index (CI) with a number afterward. p-Phenylenediamine is a known carcinogen and may cause brain damage.

Siloxanes: These compounds affect normal hormone and reproductive function. They are prevalent in hair-care products and deodorants.

Sodium lauryl sulfate: There are some studies that suggest this foaming detergent can be carcinogenic, but there's emerging evidence to the contrary. At the very least, it's an allergen and damages skin and hair follicles. This is an especially troubling side effect since it's in so many body washes and shampoos and even infants' bubble bath.

Stearalkonium chloride: This is a preservative that works as an antistatic in hair products like conditioners and gels. It's a known allergen.

Triclosan: This is an antibacterial compound added to soaps, hand sanitizers, and deodorants. It's a known skin and eye irritant and can cause hormone problems and resistance to antibiotics.

Triethanolamine: This chemical is a known irritant and allergen that has been known to trigger asthma and other negative respiratory symptoms. Unfortunately, it's also readily absorbed by your skin, a fact made more troubling by its presence in many cosmetics.

VP/VA copolymer: This is a binding compound used in skin, hair, and nail-care products. It is a known skin and respiratory irritant.

Foods as Beauty Products

So many natural and toxin-free products are available today. Some of them, however, can be pricey. There are some natural alternatives you can make yourself with food products. Baking soda cleans your hair. Coconut oil conditions your hair and your skin. Plenty of other food items can double as beauty products as well.

This is yet another way you can be in control of your toxin exposure. Making these concoctions yourself is fun, inexpensive, and gives you complete quality control. Following is one you can use every day.

Facial Cleanser

The basic idea of oil cleansing is very "European." Americans have been sloughing, using acid, and scrubbing as part of their beauty routine for years, when really all our skin needs is a little nourishment. Oil cleansing balances out the skin and remove impurities. Oil dissolves oil, while soap—meant for cleansing only—pushes dirt around on our face. Oil cleansers are now becoming very popular in high-end beauty product lines. But there is no need to spend a lot of money when all you need are two or three ingredients.

Castor oil   Tea tree oil (optional)
Olive oil

Ratios for skin type:

Oily skin: Mix 1 part castor oil with 2 parts olive oil.

Normal skin: Mix 1 part castor oil to 3 parts olive oil.

Dry skin: Mostly olive oil with a few drops of castor oil.

Acne-prone skin: Mix 1 part castor oil to 1 part olive oil with 1 or 2 drops tea tree oil.

1. In front of the sink, put a nickel-size amount of your cleansing oil mixture on a cotton ball or muslin cleansing pad and begin rubbing into your skin. It will begin to remove all the dirt and residue from your face. It even will remove your eye makeup. (If you are using tea tree oil, however, avoid the eyes.)

2. While you are rubbing the oil into your face, run the hot water and have a clean washcloth handy. When the water is hot, rinse the washcloth and blot your face, bending over to let the steam hit your skin.

3. You can repeat the process with a new washcloth until you don't see any dirt on the cloth.

Pesticide Alternative

Last, but not least, is pesticide. We are often tempted to seek and destroy the critters from the insect kingdom who invade our home. They might be creepy and crawly, but the side effects of common home pesticides are even worse. They can lead to asthma and other respiratory problems. They can also wreak havoc on all of your body's systems if they're absorbed through the skin. Again, read the warning labels on some of that stuff.

There's no need to overreact to bugs and other pests when you can keep them at bay with natural alternatives that are much less harsh. One of our favorites is another standard from Grandma and her borax solutions.

> **Borax Pesticide:** Simply sprinkle borax in tiny amounts outside around doorways to ward off mice, roaches, ants, and other insects.

GUT WISE

Warning: if you have pets and small children, they would only have to eat between 5 and 10 grams of borax for it to be a problem. Don't leave them unsupervised in the areas where you sprinkled the borax.

The Least You Need to Know

* Rid your pantry of toxic food substances and your trigger foods to take temptation out of the equation.
* Invest in good kitchen knives, a stockpot, a high-quality blender, and glass containers for food storage. If you can, splurge on a pressure cooker and/or a juicer.
* Assess your current food spending and reallocate the money to less eating out and more to stocking up on healthy gut staples for the meals you carefully plan.
* Shop the grocery-store perimeter, choosing local and organic foods whenever possible.
* Minimize your home-toxin exposure by tossing out chemical-based cleaners and personal-care products and choosing all-natural products or making your own.

Living the Healthy Gut Diet

You're armed with kitchen, pantry, and grocery store basics. You have a working knowledge of your gut and how everything you eat contributes or sabotages your health. You are now ready to live the healthy gut diet.

Part 4 helps you stick to your commitment with meal planning guidelines. We give you advice on how to prepare for traveling, holidays, and hectic schedules so you don't get off track. You also get how-to advice on eating out, cooking ahead, managing stress, and dealing with the psychology of limitation.

In addition, this part gives you the tools to forge ahead with the daily living challenges you'll face from packing a lunch for work to handling people who want you to eat birthday cake in the break room. We also arm you with foundational recipes for bone broths and fermented foods and yummy seasonal produce to help you get started.

CHAPTER 13

Lifestyle for Success

You are armed with grocery budgets, a stocked pantry and fridge, and some kitchen know-how. So now what do you do? You walk the walk. This is where so many people fail, but you will not. It's like the first day of school and everyone has their brand-new school supplies, the school floors are shiny, and students are ready to learn. A few weeks in, and some people can't find a pencil and don't really care how they did on their spelling test anymore. That will not be you. You are going to ace this.

There are several key differences between people who succeed and those who fail. People who succeed have positive attitudes, determination, support systems, and perseverance even after setbacks. You can apply these concepts to living your healthy gut diet. You got this.

In This Chapter

- Planning your meals in the short and long term
- Eating out, on-the-go, and special occasions
- Exercising and gut health
- Sleep, stress, and what it means to be "mindful"
- Coping with restriction and keeping promises to yourself

In this chapter, we set you up for success with tips for planning your meals around what feeds your digestive system, heals your gut lining, and feeds your microbiota. But food is not enough. We examine how a careful balance of exercise, rest, and introspection can contribute to optimal gut health. You also learn how to avoid the pitfalls of routine disruptions (such as travel and holidays) and the psychological challenges of dietary restrictions in a world full of temptation.

Meal Planning

A good plan is paramount to success. In Chapter 12, we gave you some tips on grocery shopping based on your meal plans and some ideas for how to build those meal plans. Think in terms of proteins and starchy and nonstarchy vegetables. Remember that dinner plate divided into three parts and think about how to fill it. It doesn't always have to be a plate. It could be a big bowl with all three major components thrown into a hearty soup. The main idea is to build meals by thinking of healthy combinations that feed your gut the fuel it needs: healthy proteins, fats, and carbohydrates in healthy proportions.

Get in touch with your produce section of your local supermarket. Learn where the organics are stocked and what's in season in your area. Learn where farmers' markets are and get to know your local growers. They're usually happy to give you tips on how to incorporate their fresh foods into your meals. You'll be surprised at the community built around healthy living that most likely exists right under your nose.

> **GUT WISE**
>
> You don't know if there's a farmers' market in your area? Here are some resources with national directories of co-op farms, local growers, and farmers' markets to find the best responsibly produced food near you: localharvest.org, ams.usda.gov/local-food-directories/farmersmarkets, and farmstandapp.com.

Plan your meals before you grocery shop, and think about the week you're going to have. We'll show you how to adjust for a busy schedule and take advantage of slow weeks to cook big batches of food that freeze well. Planning ahead will keep you on track and get you through the weeks when you don't have time to whip up meals from scratch, especially those requiring long cooking times.

Weekly Meal Plans

A lot of people make the mistake of only planning for dinners when they shop, which leaves them vulnerable to making unhealthy choices for breakfast on the go or leaves them with nothing to bring to work for lunch. Plan for all of your meals.

Breakfast can be made up of oatmeal with fruit and nuts. Or your mornings can start with smoothies packed with protein, fruit, and veggies for an all-in-one option that will make you full as well as satisfy your nutritional needs. Whole-grain breads can be used on occasion, if you can tolerate them, with a nut butter spread and fruit with yogurt on the side.

Dinner leftovers are awesome for lunch, and so are salads with added nuts, seeds (like pumpkin and chia), beans, and avocados that will satisfy volume and nutrient needs. Dinner can be made up of steamed vegetables, baked or pan sautéed meats, fermented probiotics on the side, or soups and stews made with your stocks and broths as bases. Good lunch or dinner starches are sweet potatoes and healthy whole grains in moderation.

Again, imagine that three-portion dinner plate or make big salads or soups that combine all of your nutritional needs. Get creative. Decide on your meals for the week by first considering what's in season and available at your grocery store, and plan on supplementing whatever is not in season with frozen food items.

Build your grocery list around whatever you'll need that isn't already in your pantry, fridge, or freezer. While you're looking to see what you need for meals, also take note of what staples are low and add those items to your grocery list as well. Ideally, you'll add them to your running grocery list you keep somewhere visible in your kitchen, like on your pantry or refrigerator door. We've included sample meal planners, weekly meal plans, and shopping lists in Appendix C.

Make It Ahead

Busy lifestyles can wreak havoc on your healthy intentions, but don't let a lack of time sabotage your health. Cook or prepare what you can ahead of time so when you come home from work or are busy with the demands of a morning routine, you can still pull off healthy meals.

Slow cookers can be a lifesaver for hot, home-cooked meals. You can cut up all the vegetables and meats you'll need for a soup or stew the night before and store the chopped ingredients in glass containers. It's a good idea to always keep the vegetables separate from any meat you plan to use. In the morning before going to work, you can throw all the ingredients into the slow cooker and come home to a house smelling of stew for a stress-free meal.

You can also make bone broths in a slow cooker to have your base ready for all of your soups and vegetable cooking for the week. (There's a bone broth recipe in Chapter 14.) You can even make breakfast the night before by putting chopping apples, walnuts, almond milk, and steel cut oats in a slow cooker overnight and wake up to a filling and nutritious meal to start your day.

There are other strategies you can use to make meals ahead of time. On days where you have more time, you can make extra meals or freeze your leftovers to make your own healthy lunches to go. If you want to bring your lunch to work, pack it the night before and leave yourself a note as a reminder to grab it from the refrigerator before you leave in the morning. Plan for the hectic times, and they won't be opportunities to reach for fast food or a vending machine nightmare.

If you know you want to cook a more complicated meal that involves chopping a lot of different vegetables or making a sauce that needs to cook for a long time, chop up everything you'll need the day before and store the ingredients in small containers in the refrigerator. Take meat out of the freezer the day before you'll need it and put it in the refrigerator to start thawing. These little things are like gifts to yourself, and they're much easier to do when you make a weekly plan. These small steps add up to eliminate the stress of walking in from work and thinking, "What's for dinner?"

Batch Cooking

When you're planning your weekly meals, decide which meals you can make lots of to use for some packable lunches. If you're feeling really ambitious on a Saturday or Sunday afternoon, you can put together future meals by *batch cooking*. Clearing some time to do this on a weekly or even a monthly basis will help you make your own healthy frozen meals for work or for that night you get home late and are ravenous with little time or patience to put a meal together. You can heat up your own preprepared meals in the oven or microwave the same way you might have previously reached for a commercially processed food product full of sodium and trans fat.

> **DEFINITION**
>
> **Batch cooking** is performed by multiplying a recipe to make a lot of a particular meal or dish. You store the food in batches for later use, either in casserole dishes for family meals or in individual serving sizes. "Batch cooked" meals are usually frozen.

Complicated meals that involve lots of side dishes and sauces within one meal usually don't work well with batch cooking. When reheating these kinds of meals, the different side dishes cook unevenly because they have widely varying densities and textures. The end result might be sweet potatoes that still have ice chips in them smothered in a lava-hot lentil gravy. That's no fun. The best batch cooking ideas are things like casseroles, soups, stews, quiches, and dishes that are already one incorporated piece when they're stored.

Here are some ideas of dishes that work well in batch cooking to get you started:

- Chili with chicken and beans

- Lasagna with gluten-free noodles or layers of thinly sliced zucchini, eggplant, or portobello mushrooms; and kale or spinach

- Breakfast burritos with scrambled eggs, sweet potatoes, spinach, and even lean sausage in flaxseed wraps

- Casseroles made with polenta, veggies, and chicken

- Casseroles made with squashes like spaghetti squash, with pesto or marinara sauce and added veggies

- Quiches (with or without crust) with eggs and veggies

- Any soup or stew

Here are some tips on properly storing and freezing your batches:

- Wait until the food is completely cool before freezing or subsequent condensation results in freezer burn.

- Make sure the food is as airtight in the containers as possible.

- Put dates on your containers and use within 6 months.

You can have a lot of fun coming up with dishes that pack a nutritional punch. You can sock them away and then whisk them out on a busy weeknight like a dinnertime superhero.

Eating Away from Home

Traveling for work or pleasure, spending the day at a park, dining at a restaurant, or eating at a friend's house, these are all circumstances in which we're away from our kitchens and tempted to skimp on nutrition and opt for quick, easy, or decadent.

Once your gut is healed and no longer leaky, you can indulge once in a while. But when you're on the road to superior gut health, don't be derailed by a string of small indulgences that end up reinjuring your gut lining and sending you right back to square one.

The best thing you can do to make the right choices for eating away from home is equip yourself with plans and strategies for these different situations so you won't be blindsided and cave in to sugar-, salt-, and gluten-laced pitfalls. Following are ideas for how to navigate eating away from home.

> **GUT WISE**
>
> When you know you'll be away from home for a while, pack some healthy snacks you can nibble on when you get hungry. Chapter 15's Homemade Granola Bars are a satisfying, gut-friendly snack for when you're on the go.

Order Smart

Restaurants are a part of most cultures and are often associated with special occasions, celebrations, and social events. Always saying no to meeting people at restaurants is going to make you feel ostracized and isolated. Instead, you just need to change how you order your food by choosing the healthiest options available and not being afraid to ask questions. This will involve some forethought, planning, and in some cases, calling ahead. The good news is the general public is becoming more aware of, and sensitive to, dietary restrictions, allergies, and intolerances; so many restaurants are happy to assist you. You just have to take the initiative in asking questions and choosing smart options.

Try to go to a restaurant on the early side of traditional time frames for meals so it won't be too busy. You won't feel like a burden asking for substitutions or replacements when the atmosphere in the restaurant is calm. If you feel your server is stressed out by a crowded shift with lots of tables to attend to, you're less likely to ask for what you really need.

When a meal comes with white rice or pasta, ask for portions of plain steamed vegetables instead. Ask for dressings and butter (if you can tolerate it) on the side so you can control how much seasons your meal. You can also ask for oil and vinegar on the side instead of the salty and sweet dressings often served. If there's a salad bar, go for it. When ordering fish or chicken, opt for pan-seared or baked options without breading. When the waiter first approaches your table with bread and butter, politely decline.

When attending a large catered event such as a wedding or a business gathering, call the venue ahead of time and talk with the kitchen. They are usually happy to accommodate your early requests. It gives them the opportunity to ensure their guest is happy by having time to prepare ahead rather than improvise at the spur of the moment or worse, have to decline your request because they don't have the time or alternatives to offer you.

Pack a Meal to Go

Sometimes you're on the go and healthy alternatives might not be so readily available. When you'll be traveling long distances by car, train, or bus; spending the day in a remote location; or even attending a conference where only a limited boxed lunch will be served; you'll have to bring your own food with you. Don't set yourself up for failure by not planning ahead. Packing food to go is easy and only takes a little forethought and time.

A soft insulated lunch bag and a small ice pack help you keep yogurt or tuna salad safe for several hours. Nuts are filling and give you the protein and energy surge you need.

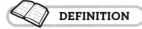

GUT WISE

As with all other "healthy" convenience food, be very careful when purchasing snacks and meal replacement bars that claim to be nutritious alternatives. Some are full of extra sugar, GMOs, and denatured ingredients that may have toxic residues like soy protein isolate. It's best to pack quick and easy snacks and meals you make yourself.

On cold days when you'll be out and about with no access to a kitchen to heat up meals, you can still enjoy comforting soups and broths. Stainless steel thermoses with *BPA*-free linings are perfect for your leftover chili, stews, soups, and even casseroles. Well-made thermoses will keep food hot for around 5 hours and cold for much longer.

DEFINITION

BPA stands for bisphenol A, a compound used in plastics and resins that can be found in food containers. The substances was labeled as safe by the U.S. Department of Health until 2010, when studies determined exposure to BPAs pose a potential risk to brain development in fetuses, infants, and small children.

You can ensure, and even extend, the cold/hot time frame for thermoses by prepping them before you load them with food. The goal is to keep foods out of the danger zone for bad bacteria growth. You want to keep cold foods at 40°F or below and hot foods above 140°F.

To prep a thermos for hot food, boil water on the stove in a small pan. While you're waiting for the water to boil, heat up the food you want to keep hot. If it's a soup or stew, heat it up until it's boiling. For all other foods, heat until it's piping hot. Remember, you're not eating it when you pack it, and it will cool down considerably even in the thermos. Once your water boils, carefully pour the hot water into the thermos, cover the thermos, and let it sit for about 4 minutes. Pour out the hot water, add your hot food, and screw the lid on tightly right away to keep in the heat.

To keep a thermos cold, open it and place it in your freezer for 10 minutes. Take the thermos out and quickly fill it with your fruit salad, homemade yogurt, gazpacho, or some other goodie you want to have cold. Even sorbets will keep for around 5 hours with this method.

Stocking a day pack with water, broth, soup, nuts, raw veggie sticks, and home-baked nonperishables will keep you energized and healthy while you venture out and about.

Other People's Homes

Going over to other people's homes for a meal is probably the most challenging part of eating away from your own kitchen. You might feel like you're insulting your hosts by not eating their food. If you know the people well, you can simply explain the diet you're trying and offer to bring a dish to share. This is especially easy to do at more casual potluck and barbecue-type gatherings.

If someone has invited you to a fancy dinner party, consider reaching out to the host ahead of time. You can explain your dietary needs and that you don't expect him or her to accommodate you. Like many other situations in life, honesty is the best policy; it doesn't have to be insulting. If you feel awkward about this situation, we understand. But imagine how your host would feel if he or she discovers you've eaten something that causes you discomfort or even pain.

In more informal situations, you can still offer to bring something to share. Be polite and explain yourself in a plain noncondescending way. If you think the dish you bring will be the only thing you'll probably be eating that evening, eat something before you go. You also might be surprised at how that conversation with your host turns into a big healthy salad as an appetizer for everyone at the party. Your decision to eat the way you do can be a conversation starter as long as you don't bring attention to yourself and make an event about you and your choices.

Holidays

Most cultures encourage an attitude of indulgence during holidays and special occasions. This can be a trying time when you're new to the healthy gut diet because you're missing the old comfort foods that have pleasant memories tied to them. The best strategy is to make healthier versions of all of these comfort foods.

Cheesecakes can be replaced by versions that use nuts. If pumpkin pie is your weakness, you can easily make one with a gluten-free crust. Did you know you can make whipped cream by putting a can of coconut milk in the refrigerator overnight? When you open the can, the fat is all right there at the top. Throw it in a cold mixing bowl with a little vanilla extract and some honey, and use it to top your pumpkin pie or other homemade baked goods.

> **GUT WISE**
>
> Chapter 15 offers numerous nourishing recipes plus some treats you'll love, including Raw Lavender and Honey "Cheesecake" and Dietitian-Approved Eggnog.

All those stuffings, gravies, and casseroles can be revised into healthy gut masterpieces. Trust us, we've done it. Birthday cakes can be made from black beans and organic dark chocolate. (Yes, that's absolutely true!) Where there's a will, there's a way. And the natural tastes of fresh produce, honey, and everything from scratch will prompt others to comment that your healthy gut versions are better than their high-sodium and vegetable oil–laden counterparts. Trust us.

During the holidays, we've "fooled" many people who didn't know something was good for them until they saw us eating it. They stopped to say, "Hey, if you're eating this, what's in it?" You can just smile and say, "Ingredients our great-grandparents would be proud of."

The Importance of Exercise

We've discussed exercise before, so we won't belabor the point too much, but we want to be certain that it's on your mind as you plan your healthy lifestyle. For optimal health, you need to incorporate some kind of exercise into your routine at least three to four times a week.

Exercise helps boost your mood, energy levels, level of digestive health, and the overall efficiency of your *metabolism*. When you make it a point to keep your body moving, you'll feel less stressed. The rush of endorphins produced by moderate to intense exercise will help combat the "fight or flight" feelings induced by chronic low-levels of stress that a lot of us have running in the back of our minds all the time. Exercise will also foster healthier sleep habits. You'll be naturally more tired at the end of the day and less likely to want to stay up too late. The quality of the sleep you get will also be greatly improved.

DEFINITION

Metabolism is the term applied to the physical and chemical processes that take place inside the cells of living organisms; basically, it's everything your body has to do to convert food into energy.

Getting Sleep and Reducing Stress

The most important thing you need to know about sleep is that without it, even your best nutrition and exercise efforts can be reversed. Like a lot of processes in our bodies, sleep is regulated by an intricate network of hormones, neurotransmitters, and organ systems.

According to the National Sleep Foundation (yes, sleep is so important that is has its own foundation), Americans are getting 20 percent less sleep nightly than they were 40 years ago. This is an epidemic with far-reaching consequences for our health. Chronic sleep deprivation can lead to metabolism issues, cardiovascular conditions, and damage to the nervous system and brain.

Aim for 8 hours a sleep at night. Plan your sleep like you would your meals. Start with when you need to wake up, and calculate 8 hours backward from that time. Then factor in the realistic amount of time you need for your bedtime routine; 8 hours should be spent entirely in bed.

That "8" is the magical number that studies show is best for most people's metabolism. Less than or more than that leads to most of us carrying around extra weight we don't need. Your needs may differ from that average 8 hours. Paying close attention to how you feel in the morning and throughout the day on more or less can help you gauge your own magical sleep number.

Like everything else in the body, balance is key. Too little sleep will disrupt your body's production of two major hormones (leptin and ghrelin) that regulate your metabolism. Less sleep cues your body to store more fat and limits your ability to regulate blood sugar. Over time, lack of sleep, actually increases the risk for obesity by 55 percent. It also affects your judgment. Being sleepy and groggy makes you less likely to do healthy things like exercise or make nutritious meals.

> **ASK THE EXPERTS**
>
> A good laugh and a long sleep are the best cures in the doctor's book.
>
> —Irish proverb

Additionally, your body takes the opportunity while you're sleeping to work on cell repair and renewal. In fact, a recent study demonstrated that the production of cells in charge of the renewal processes in your body double when you sleep. Specifically, the cells that form the protective insulation around all of your nerves and nerve tissues are produced double-time when you sleep. So make sure you turn in at a decent hour; your body depends on it.

Synch Your Gut's Sleep Clock

Your brain is home to the *suprachiasmatic nucleus* (SCN). While that may sound like a line from a Mary Poppins song, it's the fancy term for your body's master clock. It affects the rhythms of your body associated with waking and sleeping times. The master clock tries to sync up with cue based on period of light and dark in a 24-hour period. The SCN then signals the cells of the body to sync up, and this includes the cells in your gut.

Your SCN is in control of how much *melatonin* your body makes and keeping your *circadian rhythms* in check. Melatonin is a hormone that both your brain and your gut produce. In your gut, melatonin helps regulate the clock of your appetite over a 24-hour period. Melatonin production in the brain is drastically affected by your exposure to light, and the pineal gland in the brain ups its production levels when it's dark. There is also some science to suggest that gut melatonin is influenced by light exposure as well.

> **DEFINITION**
>
> The **suprachiasmatic nucleus** is a relatively small group of cells in the hypothalamus of the brain. It controls our sleep/wake cycles and circadian rhythms. **Circadian rhythms** are biological processes that are regulated by the internal clock of the SCN in roughly 24-hour long patterns. The hormone that helps modulate sleep and wake cycles is called **melatonin.**

So what does this mean for you and syncing up your SCN and your gut? Melatonin in the gut operates as a regulator of transit time. You want your gut and brain to be in sync with wake and sleep cycles so your GI tract isn't moving overtime when you need to sleep. Too little melatonin in the gut can also lead to a relaxed lower esophageal sphincter that causes acid reflux.

You can help your brain and gut prepare for healthy sleep and digestive circadian rhythms by keeping lights dim after 7 P.M., avoiding the use of electronics with brightly lit screens for 30 to 60 minutes before bedtime, and not snacking between dinner and bedtime. Wherever you sleep, it should be cool, quiet, and dark.

> **GUT WISE**
>
> Melatonin is available as a supplement to help people whose bodies aren't producing enough of the hormone to get sleepy in the evening and stay asleep all night. Doses vary widely between .2 and 20 milligrams. Everyone's needs are different. It's best to work with a health practitioner to help you find the best dosage. It's effective as a sleep aid and treatment for seasonal affective disorder and jet lag, and for resetting the circadian rhythms of people who work night shifts. It's bad news, though, if you have an autoimmune disorder. Melatonin increases the production of inflammatory cytokines. So if you have an autoimmune disease, especially rheumatoid arthritis, don't take a melatonin supplement. Research has concluded that it will worsen your condition.

Practice Mindfulness

There is a lot of talk in holistic circles these days about practicing mindfulness for better mental and physical health. So what is it? Mindfulness is a conscious effort to focus on the present moment, acknowledging how you feel emotionally, intellectually, physically, and spiritually in that moment. When we do that, we can take a kind of inventory of our stress levels and how we're reacting to them. Over time, this will make it easier to deal with stress by not holding on to tension for too long. Mindfulness can also help us appreciate when we're feeling calm and happy. A routine of mindfulness forms a pattern in our brain, so the more we do it, the easier it becomes to quiet the mind and not feel distracted and anxious.

Mindfulness is therapeutic. It can be very similar to meditation techniques. If practicing mindfulness sounds too "out there" to you, that's okay. But before you dismiss the idea outright, take a second to think about what you know about the brain-gut axis—all those connected neurons and all those microscopic bacteria communicating with our brains. Take into consideration how your bacteria respond to stress hormones. It's not too crazy of a stretch to think that consciously focusing on your body and mental states could help with better managing stress and feeling more energized and happy.

Overcoming Diet Challenges

When you're starting a nutrition regimen that requires you give up some goodies you don't want to lose, you're probably going to suffer from a psychological phenomenon known as "cognitive dissonance." This is a fancy way of labeling the discomfort you feel when you have conflicting thoughts or when you do something that contradicts your core belief. In the case of the healthy gut diet, you might really want candy, but you know at the same time it's not good for your gut bacteria and your body. Reminding yourself of the health advantages you will gain can help you overcome the challenges of your new healthy gut lifestyle.

Overcome the Psychology of Limitation

If you're really worried about giving up too many foods at once, *don't* give them up all at once. Transition gradually, taking out one bad food at a time and adding a new healthier option. Once you're well underway in your diet, try your best to eat well at least 80 to 90 percent of the time. It's better to have a positive attitude about your diet than to feel the stress of deprivation and cravings all of the time. Just don't make processed foods or other "cheating" items a regular habit. The only exception to this idea is if you've identified a food sensitivity. If you know for sure something triggers negative symptoms, find a healthier alternative to help you over the mental hump of feeling limited.

If you're trying to curb an addiction to the refined and sugary foods that pathogenic bacteria thrive on, avoiding temptation can be difficult. You might be so used to overeating these types of food that you've forgotten what true hunger feels like. The discomfort you feel when you're "hungry" is often the body's withdrawal from unhealthy food. To help replace bad habits, you have to learn what real hunger feels like and distinguish that from withdrawal.

Real hunger usually starts as a sensation below the sternum and then travel up the esophagus. If you have trouble distinguishing between real hunger and a mere craving, take stock of your environment and ask yourself why you want to eat. If it's been less than 2 or 3 hours since your last meal, if you've had a meal and are merely wanting seconds or desserts, if you're in a social setting and there's a buffet of tasty treats laid out before you, then you're probably not really hungry at all. This is another moment where practicing mindfulness can help.

> **GUT WISE**
>
> To avoid night snacking, have a healthy treat like sorbet or fruit or a healthy homemade baked good and brush your teeth shortly afterward. A clean mouth discourages most people from craving additional sweets or snacks before bed.

How you feel emotionally can have a direct effect on how well digestion operates, so it's very important to defeat the negative psychology of limitation. Your emotions affect the hormones, peptides, and neurotransmitters needed for digestion. Make sure to manage your stress and any stress you have around eating. Having a small treat and finding those alternatives to make you feel like you're not missing out can help you stay happy and healthy.

Accentuate the Positive

When you find yourself feeling down about giving up certain foods, try to spin those thoughts around. Consider everything you *get* to eat and focus on your overarching health goals.

Make a collage of positive messages about food and healthy living with pictures and quotes you find motivating and put it somewhere you can see it daily. Visualize yourself as the healthier person you want to become. Imagine all the gut discomfort or symptoms of autoimmune illness and inflammation dissipating and eventually disappearing. Imagine how happy will you be when that happens!

While it might be hard to give up certain foods you might literally be addicted to, think how much harder it is to have heart disease or chronic inflammation. Visualization exercises might sound as "out there" to you as practicing mindfulness, but there is science behind it. The patterns in the *limbic system* of your brain are the same whether you are simply visualizing an activity or actually performing the act. Visualization sets up patterns of success of failure in your brain; you might as well dream big and positive.

> **DEFINITION**
>
> The **limbic system** is a network of nerves in the brain associated with instinct and emotions. It controls our more basic feelings and instinctual drives like hunger, dominance, parenting, and sex.

How to Handle the Critics

When your brain wants to return to old habits and when you doubt your drive to succeed in cultivating a healthy lifestyle, think about what you want for yourself to drown out that negative internal voice. And there will probably be other critics, too.

It won't be uncommon for others to judge you for your choices. In a society driven by fast food, your healthy choices may make them examine their unhealthy decisions. Or they may think it's silly to give up food that makes you "happy." These are the "haters," the "Debbie Downers." Try your best to ignore them.

There seems to be an overarching view, especially in American society, of doing what makes you happy now because you could die tomorrow. This is true when we talk about living life to the fullest, but eating for a healthy gut *is* living life to the fullest. If your gut health impacts your overall well-being, then the choices you make about your gut health will lead to a happier, longer, and more productive life.

> **ASK THE EXPERTS**
>
> When we struggle with adherence to a prescribed course of action, there is a tendency to mount a defense based upon the concept of restriction. In other words: "I can't follow this because it is too restrictive." When we avoid boundaries and limits, we avoid commitment. But once we have a charted course and the necessary tools of navigation, we are liberated.
>
> —Mark Houliff, PhD, CNC, FAAIM, DCCN, Consultative Health and Nutrition

Focus on the bigger picture when people chide you for giving up junk food. Eating sweets and processed foods give a fleeting pleasure while causing long-term but slow-building damage. You're playing the long game, and long-term health goals are an investment. Most people plan for retirement and think nothing of socking money away into accounts to use much later in your life. Make the same commitment to your health.

The Least You Need to Know

- Having a plan for weekly meals will help you grocery shop effectively for optimal gut health.
- Order the healthiest options available at restaurants, pack meals and snacks to bring with you on-the-go, and find healthy alternative versions of your favorite holiday dishes.

- Exercise boosts your metabolism and improves the length and depth of your sleeping patterns.

- Your body's internal clock relies on cues, such as light and eating patterns, that you can control to improve your sleep.

- Sleep is necessary for cell renewal and health—without proper sleep the positive effects of nutrition and exercise are sabotaged.

- Overcome the negative feelings in a restricted diet by focusing on health rewards and giving yourself a treat every now and then.

CHAPTER 14

Cooking Foundational Foods

In this chapter, you learn how to make an amazing, nutrient-dense bone broth—to soothe your intestinal lining. You can use it as the base to soups, stews, and sautéed vegetables, or just sip it as a warm drink. You also learn how to make miso soup and vegetable broth for the times you're not in the mood for animal protein.

We show you how to make your own probiotic-rich fermented foods like yogurt, kefir, and vegetables. We recommend using organic ingredients in all our foundational recipes. Broths and fermented foods will promote a healthier microbiota and get you well on the way to optimal gut health.

In This Chapter

- The power of bone broths
- Vegetables broth and miso
- Fermented dairy you can make yourself
- Fermented vegetables

Gut-Soothing Broths

Bone broths have long been revered all over the world for their healing properties. They are particularly helpful for maintaining gut health. Bone broth is incredibly healthy and inexpensive way to add nutrients to your diet, and it beats the store-bought version by a landslide. Bone broths provide nourishment for the intestine's enterocytes, while they calm inflammation in the GI tract.

There's actually science behind our mothers and grandmothers pushing the stuff on us when we're sick. And while it's true that chicken bone broth can boost immune function and ease congestion, turns out it's good for us all the time. All those bioavailable amino acids, collagen, and *gelatin* are the building blocks of life.

> **DEFINITION**
>
> **Gelatin** is a water-soluble protein produced from collagen. It's very soothing to the gut.

Bone broths that begin with homemade, organic ingredients work wonders for the gut. The store-bought versions are never the same. In fact, they often contain monosodium glutamate (MSG, an unhealthful salt) and are overly processed. If you've never had real bone broth before and you've had a lot of gut issues and overall inflammatory problems, start with homemade bone broth from organic, pasture-raised chicken, as it's gentlest on the stomach and small intestine.

The most important ingredient for bone broth are quality, organic-sourced bones with just a little meat on them, joints, and even giblets if you're using a chicken or other fowl. For larger animal meats like lamb or beef, you can even ask a butcher to chop the larger tubular bones lengthwise so you can eat the marrow right after cooking while they're still soft. You can also strip the bones of their soft tissues as well. These gelatinous substances can be added to soups later. They are outstanding for healing the gut lining and boosting immunity.

Fermented Foods

Fermented foods are another great healing food used around the world. The probiotics and lactic acids they contain do wonders for gut health. Fermented foods are a highly bioavailable food, which means our bodies can easily absorb all of the foods' nutrients without losing something in the process or working too hard to get the good stuff. In addition to being nutritious, fermented foods help us get the good stuff from other foods while they're helping to heal an injured gut lining. They calm gut irritation and regulate transit time in the small intestine, so we can absorb nutrients better and have healthy bowel movements.

Gut-Healing Bone Broth

Bone broth provides calcium, magnesium, phosphorus, and other trace minerals that are very easy to digest and consume. When you make homemade bone broth, you also get gelatin and collagen from the bones, which have natural healing properties. Bone broth can be used at any time of the day. Drink a cup in the morning and take advantage of its gut-healing properties to start your day. Or use it in place of another broth in a recipe or as the base for any soups or stews. (Yield: about 1 gallon)

4 qt. filtered water	1 head garlic
2 lb. beef marrow, knuckle bones, or any other kinds of bones, including chicken neck/bones, fish, or *oxtail*	2 TB. raw and unfiltered apple cider vinegar
	1 tsp. unrefined sea salt, or to taste

1. In a 6-quart stock pot over high heat, combine water, beef, garlic, apple cider vinegar, and sea salt. Bring to a boil, reduce heat to medium-low, and simmer for at least 8 hours or up to 24 hours. (The longer it simmers, the better and more nutritious.)

2. Remove bones with a slotted spoon, and pour stock through a strainer lined with cheese-cloth or coffee filters over a large bowl.

3. If not using immediately, allow to cool slightly, divide into portioned glass or BPA-free plastic containers, and refrigerate for 1 week or freeze for up to 1 month.

Variation: For more flavor, roast the bones in the oven or brown them in a separate pot in coconut oil for a few minutes prior to putting them in the pot to boil. If you'd like, skim off the fat and save it for cooking. This is referred to as *tallow* and can be used in place of any cooking fats. You also can use a slow cooker to make any bone broth and adjust the recipe to fit the size of the slow cooker you have. Here's how: add the bones and other ingredients to the slow cooker (your bones should fill up about ¾ of the capacity of the cooker), and fill the cooker with water. Set heat to low, and check on it periodically. After 18 to 24 hours, you should have a nice layer of fat on top. Remove the bones, and strain the stock through a strainer lined with cheesecloth or coffee filters.

DEFINITION

Oxtail once referred to only the tail of an ox, but today it's used to refer to the tail of any cattle. When cooked for long periods, oxtail provides nutritious gelatin for stock.

Vegetable Broth

This simple vegetable broth offers a mild, neutral flavor base you can build on. Use it for soups, casseroles, and pilafs. It's delicious, nutritious, easy, and budget friendly. (Yield: about 1 gallon)

2 leeks, white and green parts, roughly chopped

2 medium white or yellow onions, roughly chopped

2 or 3 large carrots, roughly chopped

3 or 4 large stalks celery, roughly chopped

1 bulb fennel, roughly chopped

4 or 5 sprigs thyme

1 small bunch fresh parsley

1 tsp. whole peppercorns

1 bay leaf

1 TB. raw and unfiltered apple cider vinegar

Tomatoes, mushrooms, mushroom stems, and parsnips (optional)

4 qt. filtered water

1. In a 6-quart stock pot, combine leeks, white onions, carrots, celery, fennel, thyme, parsley, peppercorns, bay leaf, and apple cider vinegar. Add tomatoes, mushrooms, mushrooms stems, and parsnips (if using). Cover vegetables with enough water so you can easily stir them in the pot. (Less water means your broth will be more concentrated; more water makes a lighter-flavored broth.) Set over medium-high heat, and bring it to a boil. Reduce heat to low, and simmer for 40 to 50 minutes.

2. When you start to see bubbles around edges of the pot and a few wisps of steam on the surface, reduce heat to medium-low, and simmer for 45 minutes to 1 hour. Remove from heat.

3. Pour stock through a strainer lined with cheesecloth or coffee filters over a large bowl. Discard vegetables and herbs.

4. If not using immediately, allow to cool slightly, divide into portioned glass or BPA-free plastic containers, and refrigerate for 1 week or freeze for up to 1 month.

Variation: For more flavor, sauté the aromatic vegetables (onions, celery, carrots) in coconut oil for a few minutes before putting them in the pot to boil.

GUT WISE

When making vegetable broth, keep it simple with a very neutral flavor; you can always add spices and garlic when you're preparing a meal that contains the broth. You can add sea salt as you're cooking the meal as well. Too many commercially available broths and stocks add sodium and MSG, which are more reasons to make your own.

Miso Soup

Miso is a fermented soybean paste you can purchase in health food stores, Asian groceries, and even some larger grocery stores. It's usually in the refrigerated section next to the tofu. Miso is available with or without bonito, a fish. We like it with bonito because it adds an extra dynamic to the umami flavors. (Yield: 4 servings)

4 cups filtered water

1 sheet nori (dried seaweed), cut into bite-size squares (about $1/4$ cup)

3 or 4 TB. white miso paste

$1/2$ cup chopped green onion, green parts only

$1/4$ cup firm tofu, cubed

Sea salt (optional)

1. In a large saucepan over medium heat, bring water to a low simmer.

2. Add nori, and simmer for 5 to 7 minutes.

3. In a small bowl, whisk together white miso paste and a little hot water from the saucepan until smooth. (If there's a little nori in it, that's okay.) Add miso mixture to soup, stirring constantly to avoid lumps.

4. Add green onions and tofu to the saucepan, and cook, stirring occasionally, for 5 minutes.

5. Season with more miso or sea salt (if using), and serve hot.

GUT WISE

Miso paste been used in Asian cooking for centuries. The unpasteurized miso will give you the biggest nutritional bang for your buck because it contains live bacteria that are good for the gut. Miso is a fermented food made from soybeans and a culture starter called koji. (Koji is a culture starter used to make miso. It's made up of beneficial species of yeast, mold, and lactic acid bacteria.) Used in soup with mineral-rich seaweed, miso soup is gut-friendly comfort food at its best.

Kefir

Kefir is made by fermenting milk, just like yogurt, which turns it into a living food containing live bacteria or probiotics. Kefir is much more potent than yogurt because it is fermented with three to five times more strains of beneficial bacteria and yeast. It's rich in B vitamins for energy metabolism, calcium, magnesium, phosphorus, folate, vitamin K_2, and vitamin D. Because of the probiotics, kefir boosts the immune system, modulates the inflammatory response, and reduces allergies. Many who can't tolerate lactose can tolerate kefir because the fermenting process breaks down the lactose in the milk. (Yield: about 1 quart)

$\frac{1}{2}$ cup kefir grains

Milk (raw if possible or at least full-fat organic)

1. Place kefir grains in a sterilized, 1-quart glass jar.

2. Pour milk into the jar, leaving 1 inch at top. (The higher the fat content of milk, the creamier kefir will be. We like to use full-fat raw milk.) Leave the lid a bit loose to allow gas created during the fermentation process to escape.

3. Leave the jar out on the counter for 12 to 48 hours or until milk starts to thicken. Carefully shake it periodically to check for thickness. (If you leave it out too long, it will turn into curds and whey. Curds will be at the bottom, and whey will be the liquid that separates to the top. Save this if it happens. You can still drink it and use it to make cheese.)

4. Drink kefir plain, or use it in your favorite smoothies, dips, or dressings. Refrigerate until you're ready to use it.

GUT WISE

You can find kefir grains in the refrigerated dairy section of most health food stores. Also, warm temps will shorten the fermentation process, colder temps will lengthen the process.

Fermented Vegetables

Fermented foods enhance the nutrient content through a process called lacto-fermentation. During lacto-fermentation, beneficial bacteria are created that produce vitamins and enzymes to support digestion. Almost any vegetable can be fermented, and this is a great way to use and save your produce at the end of the season to enjoy it all year-round. All you need to create your own fermented veggies is sea salt and sterilized 32-ounce glass jars. (Yield: almost 1 quart)

2 or 3 TB. sea salt, or to taste

Raw, chopped organic vegetables to almost fill a 32-oz. glass jar

Fresh or dried herbs and spices

12 to 16 oz. filtered water

Cabbage leaves

1. Pour sea salt in the bottom of a sterilized 32-ounce glass jar. (This creates the right environment for the fermentation to take place and the probiotics, or "good bacteria," to grow.)

2. Fill the jar with chopped vegetables, herbs, and spices leaving 2 inches at the top of the jar.

3. Add water until it covers vegetables completely, leaving at least 1 inch at the top so there's room for vegetables to expand.

4. Place cabbage leaves on top of vegetables to keep them from touching the lid and to hold vegetables in place.

5. Set the jars on the counter to start the fermentation process. Every 48 hours, "burp" the jar to allow the gas to escape.

6. Test your vegetables around day 5 or 6 to see how they taste. They're usually best after about 1 week to 10 days.

7. When vegetables have reached the level of fermentation you like, refrigerate the jar for up to 9 months.

GUT WISE

You can use any combination of raw organic vegetables in this dish. Try chopped cauliflower, chopped beets, chopped carrots, chopped green beans, chopped bell peppers, sliced radishes, sliced cucumbers, chopped turnips, chopped broccoli, chopped onions, and chopped garlic. For the herbs and spices, you can try dried chile peppers, black peppercorns, bay leaves, fresh dill, fresh basil, fresh tarragon, or fresh mint. If you're feeling adventurous and up for trying a fermented veggie, try natto. Natto is made by fermenting soybeans with Bacillus subtilis. It's pungent and slimy, but it's a traditional Japanese superfood and probiotic that your gut will love.

Kimchi

Making kimchi can be a long process, but it's so worth it. Kimchi can be made in a range of flavors, from very mild to spicy. This recipe is very spicy, so to tame it a bit, reduce the gingerroot and chile flakes by half or leave them out entirely. Use organic produce if at all possible. (Yield: approximately 4 32-ounce glass jars)

1 head organic napa cabbage, shredded, a few whole leaves reserved

1 bunch organic kale, shredded

6 green onions, chopped

1 medium organic golden beet, shredded

1 medium daikon radish, shredded

1 medium organic Granny Smith apple, shredded

½ cup shredded gingerroot

3 cloves organic garlic, minced

2 large organic carrots, shredded

1 TB. ground turmeric

3 TB. chile flakes

2 TB. sea salt

1 or 2 cups filtered water

3 TB. raw and unfiltered apple cider vinegar

Raw local honey or grade B maple syrup

1 or 2 probiotics capsules as "starters" (optional)

1. In a large bowl, combine napa cabbage, kale, green onions, golden beet, daikon radish, Granny Smith apple, gingerroot, garlic, carrots, turmeric, chile flakes, and sea salt. Massage ingredients together for a few minutes until they all are soft and juicy. Pack mixture into several large glass jars, pressing mixture into the jar, but leaving some room at the top.

2. In a small bowl, combine water, apple cider vinegar, and honey. Pour about ½ cup into each jar, leaving only 1 or 2 inches for vegetables to expand. (If you need additional liquid, fill with more water.)

3. Use a piece of cabbage under the lid to keep the liquids from the metal, and tightly screw on the lid of each jar.

4. Shake well, and store in a dark, cool place for 3 or 4 days, weeks, or up to 1 month. Shake jars daily. (The longer you keep them, the stronger the flavors.) Open the jars, taste kimchi, and adjust for seasonings. If it's too sour, add 1 to 3 tablespoons more honey. When kimchi has reached a flavor you enjoy, store in the refrigerator for several weeks if not months.

GUT WISE

Enjoy kimchi as a salad, sandwich topping, mixed into gluten-free grain dishes, or by the spoonful. Eat it daily to help improve digestion and reduce inflammation.

Homemade Yogurt

Yogurt is a mixture of fat, whey, casein protein, and beneficial bacteria. It's very high in protein, probiotics, vitamins, and minerals, and it can help restore healthy flora in your gut. Making your own yogurt allows you to control the quality of the ingredients. You will need good-quality whole milk or cream and bacterial starter (available online or at health food stores in the dairy section). Good bacterial starters include GI ProStart, Cultures for Health, or Custom Probiotics. You also can use a bit of leftover yogurt from a previous batch or a good-quality store-bought full-fat plain yogurt. (Yield: about 1 quart)

4 cups whole milk or cream (raw, organic, or grass-fed are best)

Powdered bacterial yogurt starter, or $\frac{1}{4}$ cup good-quality plain full-fat yogurt with live active cultures and $\frac{1}{2}$ cup whole milk

1. Sterilize your glass jars by running them through a dishwasher or boiling them in hot water. (You can use $\frac{1}{2}$ pint or 1 pint jars, depending on how you like to store them for convenient eating later. You'll also need a larger jar for mixing.) If you do not sterilize your jars, the bacteria can take over your starter. When this happens, the end result will not taste like yogurt.

2. In a large saucepan over medium-low heat, heat milk, stirring often so you don't scorch milk. Bring milk to 180°F on a thermometer or until it starts bubbling around the edge of the pan.

3. Before adding starter, cool milk slightly to room temperature. (This process can be sped up by pouring milk into the jars and setting them in cool water.) This step is very important because if milk is too hot, it will kill all bacteria in starter.

4. If you are using a powdered starter, follow the instructions on the package for quantities. It's easier mixed in one sterilized, large $\frac{1}{2}$-gallon jar than separating. If using leftover yogurt, prepare a paste using $\frac{1}{2}$ cup milk and $\frac{1}{4}$ cup leftover yogurt, and add it to cooled milk.

5. Put the lids on the jars, close tightly, and place in the oven with the door closed and the light on for 24 hours. Yogurt will still be runny when you remove it from the oven, but it will thicken as it cools. (Yogurt can sometimes be more liquid than store-bought, but the taste will be great! The quality and strength of starter, length of time, and temperature during the fermentation process all can affect the thickness.)

6. Refrigerate yogurt until ready to use.

YOU ARE WHAT YOU EAT

If you consistently have trouble with cow's milk products, try raw milk from a reliable source or switch up the animal source. Goat and sheep produce milk with a difference kind of casein that more people can tolerate. You may also want to try sour cream as your fermented food instead. Cream has only trace amount of casein because it's mostly fat. Opt for full-fat organic sour cream and keep in mind that it will only retain its probiotic benefits as long as it's cold. You can make creamy sauces with it, but then you kill all the bacteria in it.

The Least You Need to Know

- Cooking for yourself is a great joy that ensures responsibly sourced ingredients for the best nutrient-dense foods.
- Bone broths are outstanding sources of amino acids that promote immune system function as well as gut lining healing.
- Fermented foods are natural sources of bioavailable probiotics that will balance your gut microbiota.
- Fermented dairy may be tolerated even by those who have problems with other forms of dairy.

CHAPTER 15

Healthy Gut Recipes

You have the foundational recipes down now. You can incorporate the broths into your daily meals as a cooking agent or the base for a soup or stew. You can also supplement any meal with fermented foods.

In this chapter, you expand your healthy gut know-how to include fresh, healthy foods. Building meals around what's in-season, organic, and local boosts your nutrient intake and ensures freshness and quality. Supplement your meals with frozen fruits and vegetables, gluten-free or organic whole grains, and your foundational broths and fermented foods, and you'll have a well-rounded, delicious, gut-healing menu.

In This Chapter

- Cooking for a healthy gut
- Nutrient-dense dishes
- Delicious and gut-friendly recipes

Sunday Brunch Bowl with Truffled Polenta

This brunch bowl incorporates white truffle oil and smoked buffalo mozzarella. When asparagus is in season, this is the only brunch recipe you need. We use farm-fresh eggs and love the runny yolk. Crumbled pastured local bacon completes this tasty dish. (Yield: 4 servings)

$4^1/_2$ cups vegetable or chicken broth

$^1/_4$ tsp. sea salt, or to taste

1 cup polenta

1 cup smoked buffalo mozzarella cheese, chopped

2 TB. olive oil

1 clove garlic

1 bunch green onions

$^1/_2$ medium white onion (or your favorite), chopped

1 bunch asparagus, chopped

1 TB. fresh rosemary, chopped

Fresh ground pepper

4 cups water (optional)

1 tsp. white or apple cider vinegar (optional)

4 farm fresh eggs (optional)

$^1/_2$ lb. pastured bacon, cooked and crumbled

Truffle salt or truffle olive oil

1. In a 3-quart saucepan over high heat, bring 4 cups vegetable broth to a boil.

2. Add sea salt, and slowly whisk in polenta.

3. Reduce heat to low, add smoked buffalo mozzarella cheese, and continue to whisk until mixture starts to thicken. Cover and cook, uncovering occasionally to stir and scrape the side of the pan, for 30 to 40 minutes.

4. Meanwhile, in medium skillet over medium heat, heat olive oil. Add garlic, and cook, stirring for 2 minutes, or until fragrant.

5. Add remaining $^1/_2$ cup vegetable broth, green onions, white onion, and asparagus. Cover and cook for 10 minutes, stirring halfway through.

6. Remove from heat, and season with rosemary and pepper.

7. If including eggs in your polenta, in a $1^1/_2$-quart saucepan over high heat, bring water and white vinegar to a boil. Reduce heat to low, and carefully crack eggs into water. Cook for $3^1/_2$ minutes, remove eggs from water using a slotted spoon, and set aside.

8. To assemble, spoon polenta into shallow serving bowls. Top each serving with vegetable mixture, crumbled bacon, and a poached egg (if using). Season with truffle salt, and serve.

Sausage and Green Chile Frittata

This recipe is very easy to prepare, and if you have a cast-iron skillet, it's even better. If not, you can make it in a pie pan after the stovetop cooking. (Yield: 6 servings)

1 TB. grass-fed butter

$\frac{1}{2}$ cup diced white or yellow onion

$\frac{1}{2}$ lb. organic sweet Italian sausage

7 farm fresh eggs

$\frac{1}{2}$ cup unsweetened coconut milk

$\frac{1}{2}$ cup shredded grass-fed cheese (any variety)

1 (4-oz.) can chopped green chilies, drained

1 cup diced tomatoes

1. Preheat the oven to 350°F.

2. In a cast-iron skillet over medium heat, melt butter. Add white onion and Italian sausage, and cook, stirring regularly to ensure sausage cooks through, for 10 minutes or until browned.

3. In a large bowl, combine eggs, coconut milk, and cheese. Set aside.

4. Add green chilies and tomatoes to the skillet, cover with egg mixture, and stir until combined.

5. Place skillet in the oven, and bake for 25 minutes or until the center is set. Serve hot.

Grilled Garlic Scapes

We love farmers' markets, and garlic scapes are in abundance in the spring. Scapes are the shoots that come out of the ground from the hardneck variety of garlic. They are a vegetable, aromatic, and herb all in one. If you come across them in the spring, grab a handful and give them a try. This is one of our favorite ways to incorporate them! (Yield: about 1 cup)

1 bunch garlic scapes

2 TB. extra-virgin olive oil

Sea salt

Fresh ground pepper

1. Toss garlic scapes in extra-virgin olive oil, and season with sea salt and pepper.

2. Char over a hot grill, and serve hot. Add to salads, and serve as a complement to whatever you were planning for breakfast, lunch, or dinner.

Moroccan Quinoa Salad

You can make this salad in advance and portion it out for easy lunches during the week. Then all you have to do before a busy day is grab-and-go. Dried apricots, fresh mint, and pea shoots make this salad especially delicious. (Yield: 3 or 4 servings)

1 head romaine lettuce, chopped

1 cup Bibb lettuce, chopped

$\frac{1}{4}$ cup fresh mint, chopped

$\frac{3}{4}$ cup quinoa

$1\frac{1}{2}$ cups water

$\frac{1}{4}$ cup slivered almonds

$\frac{1}{4}$ cup dried apricots, chopped

Pea shoots

1. In a large bowl, combine romaine lettuce, Bibb lettuce, and mint.

2. Rinse quinoa thoroughly in a fine-meshed sieve, and place in a $1\frac{1}{2}$-quart saucepan. Add water, set over high heat, and bring to a boil. Reduce heat to medium-low, cover, and simmer for about 20 minutes or until all water is absorbed. Fluff with a fork.

3. Meanwhile, preheat the oven to 350°F.

4. Place almonds in a single layer on a rimmed baking sheet, and toast for about 10 minutes.

5. Layer cooked quinoa, toasted almonds, and apricots over salad, top with pea shoots, and serve.

GUT WISE

Quinoa is a seed that's been cultivated in the Andean regions of Peru and Bolivia for nearly 7,000 years. It's a great source of healthy fats, protein, and carbs.

Grilled Pattypan Pizzas

This is a very simple summer recipe for the grill. The "crust" is nothing more than a pattypan squash found from a local farmers' market. And remember, you can omit the cheese if you are sensitive to dairy. (Yield: 4 servings)

2 pattypan squash

2 TB. 100 percent extra-virgin olive oil

½ cup marinara sauce

1 tomato, sliced

1 cup shredded provolone cheese (optional)

Freshly shredded Parmesan cheese (optional)

Fresh basil

1. Preheat the grill to medium. Preheat the broiler.

2. Halve each pattypan squash horizontally to make 4 round slices. Scoop out the seeds.

3. Brush with squash with extra-virgin olive oil, place on the grill, and cook for 15 minutes, turning halfway through.

4. Spoon 2 tablespoons marinara sauce on each slice. Top each slice with 1 piece of tomato and ¼ cup provolone cheese (if using), and sprinkle with Parmesan cheese (if using).

5. Transfer to the oven, and broil high for 8 to 10 minutes or until cheese is bubbly.

6. Top with fresh basil, and serve.

GUT WISE

Make sure the marinara sauce has quality ingredients, including olive oil. Stay away from corn syrup, vegetable oil, and soybean oil in marinara sauces.

Easy Weeknight Turkey Burgers

If you need an easy weeknight dinner that's healthy *and* kid friendly, these burgers are an ideal choice. The sun-dried tomatoes and red onion stand up well to the feta. The burgers can be served on gluten-free buns or on beds of spinach. (Yield: 4 servings)

1 lb. ground turkey	1 clove garlic, minced
$\frac{1}{2}$ medium red onion	Sea salt
$\frac{1}{2}$ cup sun-dried tomatoes, chopped	Pepper
$\frac{1}{2}$ cup feta cheese, crumbled	Roasted red peppers
$\frac{1}{2}$ cup plain Greek yogurt	Spinach
Juice from $\frac{1}{2}$ medium lemon	

1. Preheat the grill to medium.

2. In a large bowl, combine turkey, red onion, sun-dried tomatoes, and feta cheese. Form mixture into 4 equal-size patties.

3. Grill burgers for 3 to 5 minutes on each side until they reach your desired level (medium-rare to well-done), or pan-fry over medium heat for 3 to 5 minutes per side or until well done.

4. In a small bowl, combine Greek yogurt, lemon juice, garlic, sea salt, and pepper.

5. Top burgers with roasted red peppers and spinach, and finish with a drizzle of yogurt sauce. Serve on top of a salad, or enjoy with gluten-free buns.

GUT WISE

In addition to being delicious, garlic also has proven immune boosting power. According to a 2001 study published in the U.S. National Library of Medicine, if you have a cold, increasing your intake of garlic can shorten the duration of the cold by 70 percent. It also lowers blood pressure and cholesterol levels and is an antioxidant. It truly is a superfood.

Avocado, Sun-Dried Tomato, and Goat Cheese Burgers

We've tried all kinds of burgers, but these stuffed burgers really hit the spot. They'll be a fan favorite at summer barbecues. (Yield: 4 servings)

3 lb. grass-fed ground beef

2 TB. sun-dried tomatoes, chopped

2¼ cup goat cheese, crumbled

½ medium Hass avocado, peeled, seeded, and chopped

2 TB. extra-virgin olive oil

Sea salt

Fresh cracked pepper

Lettuce, tomato, and onion for garnish

1. Preheat the grill to medium.

2. Form ground beef into 4 equal-size patties.

3. Make small pockets in patties, and stuff with sun-dried tomatoes, goat cheese, and Hass avocado.

4. Brush burgers with extra-virgin olive oil, and season with sea salt and pepper.

5. Place burgers on the grill, and grill one side for about 3 minutes or until lightly browned and charred.

6. Flip over burgers, and grill the other side for about 4 minutes (for medium) or to your desired level of doneness.

7. Serve burgers on gluten-free buns, or "naked" with lettuce, tomato, and onion.

 YOU ARE WHAT YOU EAT

Sun-dried tomatoes are packed with lycopene, a powerful antioxidant. While lycopene is in all tomatoes, it is more concentrated and bioavailable in sun-dried tomatoes than raw tomatoes.

Summer Sunshine Bowls

Coriander, cumin, and turmeric give this bowl its delicious flavor. It's the perfect "throw-together" meal you can make at the last minute and still get your greens, protein, and healthy carbs. (Yield: 2 servings)

½ cup quinoa

3 tsp. extra-virgin olive oil

1 cup vegetable or bone broth

1 clove garlic, minced

1 cup cooked chickpeas

1 cup purple cauliflower, chopped

½ tsp. coriander

½ tsp. cumin

½ tsp. turmeric

¼ tsp. crushed red pepper flakes

2 TB. chopped fresh cilantro

2 farm fresh eggs (optional)

1 cup baby kale or any fresh greens

1 cup cherry tomatoes, halved

1. Rinse quinoa thoroughly with a fine-meshed sieve.

2. In a Dutch oven or large saucepan over medium heat, heat 1 teaspoon extra-virgin olive oil. Add quinoa, and toast for 1 minute or until nutty and fragrant.

3. Add vegetable broth, and bring to a boil. Reduce heat to low, and simmer for 15 minutes until quinoa absorbs liquid. Fluff with a fork.

4. In a sauté pan over medium heat, heat remaining 2 teaspoons extra-virgin olive oil. Add garlic, and cook for about 1 minute or until aromatic.

5. Add chickpeas, purple cauliflower, coriander, cumin, turmeric, and crushed red pepper flakes. Cook for 5 to 10 minutes or until cauliflower is crunchy but not cooked through.

6. Add quinoa and cilantro.

7. If you want eggs to top your dish, spray a frying pan or skillet with coconut or olive oil cooking spray and set over medium heat. Crack eggs into the pan, and cook for about 4 minutes or until white is no longer translucent and yolk reaches your desired texture. Remove from heat.

8. Layer baby kale, quinoa mixture, cherry tomatoes, and cooked eggs (if using) in 2 bowls, and serve hot.

GUT WISE

Turmeric boosts your immune system function. In addition to cooking with it, you can also take it as a supplement.

Curried Sweet Potatoes, Chickpeas, and Spinach with Coconut Rice

This dish is chock full of iron and protein and is very easy to make. It's a nutritious and filling weeknight meal that also makes great leftovers. (Yield: 4 servings)

6 cups vegetable broth

1 large raw sweet potato, peeled and chopped into $^3/_4$-in. squares

2 cups cooked chickpeas or 1 (15-oz.) can Eden organic garbanzo beans, rinsed and drained

2 cups fresh baby spinach

$^1/_2$ cup fresh cilantro, chopped

$^1/_2$ tsp. sea salt

1 tsp. coriander

1 tsp. curry powder

$^1/_2$ tsp. cumin

$^1/_2$ tsp. garam masala

2 cups whole brown rice or quinoa

1 (13-oz.) can organic full-fat coconut milk

1 tsp. Thai red chile paste

1. In a medium saucepan over medium heat, simmer 2 cups vegetable broth and sweet potatoes for about 15 minutes or until sweet potatoes begin to soften.

2. Add chickpeas and baby spinach, and stir until spinach wilts.

3. Add cilantro, sea salt, coriander, curry powder, cumin, and garam masala, and simmer for 10 minutes or until mixture reaches your desired thickness.

4. Meanwhile, in a medium saucepan, cook brown rice in remaining 4 cups vegetable broth according to package directions.

5. In a small saucepan over medium heat, heat coconut milk until simmering. Add Thai red chile paste, reduce heat to low, and keep warm.

6. When rice is cooked, pour in coconut chile sauce, and stir well.

7. Dish out a big bowl of coconut rice, spoon sweet potato mixture over top, and serve hot.

Turnip, Leek, and Cauliflower Bisque

This flavorful vegetable soup is guaranteed to warm you from the inside out. (Yield: 1½ quarts)

4 cups vegetable broth

3 or 4 medium leeks, cleaned, dark green sections removed, and chopped

Sea salt

Freshly cracked pepper

3 large turnips, purple skins peeled

1 medium head cauliflower, trimmed and cut into florets

½ cup organic white cooking wine

3 cups unsweetened almond milk

½ tsp. dried thyme

1 TB. fresh chives, snipped or chopped

1. In a 6-quart saucepan over medium heat, heat 1½ cups vegetable broth.

2. Add leeks and a heavy pinch of sea salt and pepper, increase heat to medium-high, and sweat leeks for 5 minutes.

3. Reduce heat to medium-low, and cook, stirring occasionally, for about 25 minutes or until leeks are tender.

4. Add turnips, cauliflower, remaining 2½ cups vegetable broth, and white wine. Increase heat to medium-high, and bring to a boil.

5. Reduce heat to low, cover, and gently simmer for about 35 minutes or until turnips and cauliflower are soft.

6. Remove from heat, and purée mixture in a blender until smooth.

7. Stir in almond milk, and add thyme. Taste and adjust seasoning if desired.

8. Sprinkle with chives, and serve.

GUT WISE

You can substitute soy or hemp milk for the almond milk, but almond tastes best in this recipe.

Chicken Piccata

This chicken dish is a hearty, protein-rich meal that's perfect for a brisk day. (Yield: 4 servings)

1 pkg. chicken cutlets
   (approximately 4)
Sea salt
Fresh ground pepper
Freshly grated Parmesan cheese
6 TB. grass-fed butter

3 TB. olive oil
2 small lemons
½ cup chicken stock
¼ cup capers, rinsed
⅓ cup fresh parsley, chopped

1. Season chicken cutlets with sea salt and pepper, and dredge in Parmesan cheese.

2. In a large stainless-steel skillet over medium-high heat, melt 2 tablespoons butter and 3 tablespoons olive oil. Add chicken, and brown on both sides for about 3 or 4 minutes per side. Transfer chicken to a plate.

3. Slice 1 lemon, add it to the skillet, and brown for 2 minutes.

4. Transfer lemon slices to top of chicken.

5. Set skillet heat to medium, and melt remaining 4 tablespoons butter. Add chicken stock, juice of remaining lemon, and capers, and stir, scraping the side of the pan.

6. Bring to a boil, reduce heat to medium, return chicken to the pan, and coat chicken in sauce.

7. Cook for 5 minutes, transfer chicken to a plate, garnish with parsley, and serve.

Homemade Granola Bars

These hearty granola bars will satisfy you when you're on the go. (Yield: 8 bars)

10 pitted Medjool dates

1 cup gluten-free rolled oats

1/2 cup chopped raw sliced almonds

1/4 cup raw honey

1/4 cup natural peanut butter

Enjoy Life chocolate chips or cacao nibs

1. In food processor fitted with a metal chopping blade, process Medjool dates until they form a ball.

2. Transfer dates to a large bowl, add rolled oats and almonds, and set aside.

3. In a small saucepan over medium heat, heat honey and peanut butter. Pour mixture over dates, oats, and almonds, and stir until combined.

4. Press batter into an 8×8 baking dish lined with plastic wrap, sprinkle some Enjoy Life chocolate chips over the top, and refrigerate for 20 minutes.

5. Cut into bars, and store in an airtight container for up to 7 days.

Red, White, and Blue Chia Seed Pudding

Chia seeds are a superfood full of healthy fats and soluble fiber, which are fabulous for the digestive system. (Yield: 1 serving)

1 cup plus 1 tablespoon strawberries, chopped

2 TB. chia seeds

1 cup plain Greek yogurt or kefir

2 TB. unsweetened shredded coconut

1 cup blueberries (plus a few extra for topping)

1. In a blender, combine 1 cup strawberries and 1 tablespoon chia seeds for 1 minute.

2. Transfer mixture to a glass jar or drinking glass, top with remaining 1 tablespoon strawberries, and freeze for 10 minutes.

3. Add Greek yogurt, top with coconut, and freeze for 10 more minutes.

4. In the clean blender, combine 1 cup blueberries and remaining 1 tablespoon chia seeds for 1 minute.

5. Pour blueberry mixture over Greek yogurt, top with remaining blueberries, and serve.

Raw Lavender and Honey "Cheesecake"

This flavorful dessert is vegan, raw, gluten free, and dairy free. The texture and flavor are amazing, and it's filled with healthy fats and protein. Raw local honey drizzled on top gives it sweetness without being too overpowering. You can even make it in silicone muffin pans to keep portions in check. (Yield: 12 servings)

2 cups raw cashews

1 cup raw almonds

1 cup (about 10) pitted dates

$\frac{1}{2}$ cup extra-virgin cold-pressed organic coconut oil

Sea salt

$\frac{1}{2}$ cup organic full-fat coconut milk

$\frac{1}{2}$ cup maple syrup

1 tsp. pure vanilla extract

Lavender-infused honey

$\frac{1}{2}$ cup unsweetened shredded coconut

1. The night before preparing recipe, cover cashews with water, and soak overnight or for 8 to 12 hours. Rinse, drain, and set aside.

2. The next day, lightly grease 12 muffin cups with coconut oil cooking spray or butter.

3. In a food processor, blend almonds, dates, $\frac{1}{4}$ cup extra-virgin coconut oil, and sea salt until mixture begins to clump. Press crust mixture evenly among 12 lightly greased muffin pan cups.

4. In a blender, combine cashews, coconut milk, remaining $\frac{1}{4}$ cup extra-virgin coconut oil, maple syrup, and vanilla extract until completely smooth. Pour over crust in muffin cups.

5. Freeze for 1 hour.

6. Top with lavender-infused honey and shredded coconut, and serve.

GUT WISE

To infuse honey with lavender, simply put lavender buds into honey and let it sit for 24 to 48 hours.

Dietitian-Approved Eggnog

No need to miss out on one of the holiday season's greatest treats with this healthier eggnog made without loads of sugar. It's even better when it's made a day or more in advance of your party. (Yield: 6 servings)

2 cups raw or organic pasteurized milk

2 cups organic pasteurized cream

8 farm fresh eggs

2 tsp. vanilla extract

2 tsp. ground cinnamon

2 tsp. pumpkin pie spice or allspice

4 TB. real maple syrup

Bourbon or rum to taste

1. In a blender, combine milk, cream, eggs, vanilla extract, cinnamon, pumpkin pie spice, maple syrup, and bourbon.

2. Refrigerate, and serve cold.

The Least You Need to Know

- Include fresh, whole foods with as many organic ingredients as possible in your daily meals.
- Build meals around in-season, organic, and local produce to get the most nutrients.
- Supplement meals with frozen vegetables when fresh isn't available.
- Incorporate gut-healing bone broths and fermented foods into your menu.

PART

5

Finding a Healthy Gut Balance

Now that you know the rationale behind the healthy gut diet and how to move forward with grocery shopping and cooking amazing meals, it's time to talk about finding a balance you can sustain.

In this part, we let you know what to expect and prepare for as you move forward. You learn about the challenges of detoxing your body and dealing with relapses. We also show you how to deal with temptation and successfully reintroduce former trigger foods.

We help you learn to troubleshoot your gut symptoms and make adjustments by giving you specific tools to track your progress. A skin sensitivity test enables you to predict problems with the reintroduction of trigger foods. Food and lifestyle diaries help you keep tabs on what influences your personal gut health.

CHAPTER 16

Giving the Diet Time

Weaning yourself off processed foods and triggers that have built up in your system will most likely cause you some temporary discomfort. We just want to be up front about that. And the unpleasant stuff might not be all psychological. You'll probably feel it physically as well. As bad bacteria die off in your gut and you flush toxins out of their hiding places in your body's tissues, you might feel lousy. Take heart. This is the prelude to feeling amazing.

In this chapter, we explain detox symptoms and help you cope. We also discuss what to do if your GI symptoms keep persisting even though you're being "good." There are some pesky underlying problems that need professional guidance, and we outline what are some of those conditions. Most excitingly, we cover the long-term health benefits of the healthy gut diet, including disease prevention and reversal.

In This Chapter

* Common side effects of detox
* How to deal with persistent GI symptoms
* When to seek professional help
* Health benefits of the healthy gut diet

What to Expect

People think nothing of expecting withdrawal symptoms when someone gives up drugs. But they don't make this connection with giving up processed and unhealthy foods. Your body may have become addicted to these foods. Additionally, your other habits and toxin exposure over time can also induce some unpleasant symptoms while you detox.

It's normal to experience some discomfort while your body flushes out so many built-up toxins and repairs its cells. Your body is always engaged in these processes, even under the best of circumstances. The healthy gut diet just streamlines the process and makes it easier for your body. Decreasing the toxic load you've been carrying will help achieve gut homeostasis and maintain a healthy GI tract as you reestablish your healthy microbiota. Detoxing initially overloads your system, but it then gives your liver and immune system a much-needed break to heal and repair.

The Symptoms of Detoxification

You can minimize the symptoms of detoxing by gradually cutting out unhealthy foods and exchanging them for healthy options. This approach works well for some people and is more like weaning than quitting "cold turkey." On the other hand, the all-or-nothing mentality can also stop people from prolonging a period of indulgence in all the sugars, caffeine, processed foods, and unhealthy fats and carbs they crave. Clearing out the cabinets, trashing the triggers, and having only healthy options on hand can help you stay focused and on track.

Whichever route you decide will be best for you is still a step toward optimal gut health. Just be aware that giving up the foods that overstimulate the pleasure receptors in the brain, and your body's systems in general, might have some short-term, short-lived negative consequences.

Common detox symptoms include fatigue (careful with this one—it often means you're simply not taking in enough calories), headaches, achy joints, irritability, craving for sweet and salty foods, nausea, change in bowel habits (diarrhea or constipation), tremors, anxiety, brain fog (often indicates a lack of nutrients—track your food and make sure you're getting what you need), depression, itchiness, rashes, acne, and other skin irritation.

The severity of these symptoms will depend on your previous eating habits and any underlying conditions you have. Any nasty symptoms usually last between a few days and 2 weeks at most. Really severe and prolonged detox symptoms are rare but can occur in people with autism and schizophrenia when casein and gluten are taken out of their diets because their low stomach acid and imbalanced gut bacteria converted those proteins into opiate-like substances. So removing dairy and gluten from their diets is really like taking drugs away from an addict.

Success Story

S. Jane Gari

My own detox story is pretty typical of someone addicted to dairy and gluten. I was a lacto-ovo vegetarian and got a lot of my protein from milk products. Cheese, bread, and the fake meat alternatives laced with MSG and soy protein isolate were my comfort foods of choice. After eating this way for several years, I started to notice swelling and stiffness in my neck vertebrae, fingers, feet, and knees. The symptoms would come and go with up to 3 months in between flare-ups.

When I was finally diagnosed with rheumatoid and psoriatic arthritis, I just figured I'd take the pills the doctors told me to and go about life with some mild discomfort and fatigue from time to time. After a major stomach bleed caused by those meds, I decided to get radical about nutrition and start researching what was really going on in my body.

Overly processed wheat, low-fat processed dairy, and vegetarian "junk food" marketed as protein made up a huge part of my diet. But I gave them all up—no transitioning. Once I knew how those foods were damaging my gut and brain and causing floods of zonulin and making my gut leaky, I just couldn't look at them the same way. That doesn't mean the "cold-turkey" method was easy. My symptoms were very prolonged because my system was so clogged with toxins.

For 5 weeks I felt like I had a bad case of the flu. In short, I was miserable. I ate nothing but brown rice, quinoa, fermented soy (miso and tempeh), and as many vegetables as I could. I had to keep upping my calories and felt like I was on a baby's eating schedule. More than once I thought about caving and just trying a different medication in the hopes the side effects would be manageable.

After that 5-week mark, something amazing happened. I woke up one morning and for the first time in years I could make a fist. My fingers weren't swollen. I could wear my wedding ring without having to ice my fingers and coax it on with lotion. I cried with relief. The diet was working. I never looked back. It's been 7 years now.

These days I can tolerate fermented dairy and have reintroduced meat proteins like fish and bone broths into my diet with wonderful results. The only flare-ups of autoimmunity come in times of serious stress when I don't get enough sleep or exercise. However, once I get back on track, the inflammation subsides. Detox symptoms aren't pleasant; there's no way around them, only through them. But once you're through, you will feel like a new person.

Another part of detox is referred to as "bacteria die-off." When you take probiotic supplements and eat probiotic foods, the good bacteria recolonize your gut and kill off large portions of the pathogenic bacteria that had taken over your gut. When those bad bacteria die off, they release toxins.

As gross as it might sound, detoxing can temporarily turn your gut into a battlefield strewn with dead bodies. But take heart; you're winning the war. You just need to be patient while all of your internal mechanisms are clearing out the carnage. This has some short-term unpleasant side effects, such as fatigue, skin rashes, or a worsening of symptoms you endured before detoxing. If the die-off symptoms are really hard for you to deal with, you can decrease your probiotic dose or eat smaller portions of probiotic foods. If you've been suffering from long-term illnesses with uncomfortable symptoms, you can ease into a probiotic regimen and slowly increase your daily intake. This gradual introduction of probiotics will lessen the severity of die-off symptoms.

Digestion Discomfort: What's Normal?

While you're transitioning to a healthy gut diet, you might experience some detox symptoms, and you might have other symptoms that aren't necessarily a release of toxins but your body just adjusting to the new fuel you're feeding it. It's common to have some GI tract discomfort if your body wasn't used to eating so many healthy fats, leafy greens, and vegetables in general.

An increase in gas and bloating is a normal side effect of a sudden uptick in daily fruits and veggies. Give it a few days for your body to adjust. If the bloating and gas continue and are uncomfortable, and your belly gets really distended, then try smaller portions. Remember to keep a food diary, so you can track which vegetables and fruits are the culprits. To make it easier for yourself, only have one vegetable or fruit at a time and not a mix of several different kinds. As you progress, you can spice things up with more variety, but limitation and tracking are key to troubleshooting.

A change in bowel habits is common when you switch up your diet. It's completely logical when you think about it. An input change is going to cause an output change. Diarrhea is a common side effect of a sudden uptick in fruits and veggies, especially if you didn't eat a lot of them before. This should subside in 2 or 3 days. Constipation is a rarer reaction to a more nutrient-dense diet, but a sudden increase in fiber can cause this in some people. Make sure you're drinking plenty of water between meals and your transit time should regulate itself within a couple of days.

Success Story

Client of Wendie Schneider, RDN, LD, MBA

For as long as she could remember, one of my clients suffered with IBS and heartburn. As the years went by, it worsened. By the time she graduated college and entered the professional world, she suffered from a weakened immune system and low energy levels. As she entered her 30s, she was diagnosed with hypothyroidism, chronic fatigue, and chronic allergies. In her late 30s, she had her first child and developed severe food allergies and eczema.

Many doctors attempted to treat her with antibiotics, steroids, and various other drugs. She sought the help of an integrative physician and came to see me for help with her diet. She had gut hyperpermeability ("leaky gut") from years of strong antibiotics, steroids, and iron supplements from her pregnancy.

She started on my Gut Healing Program that included probiotics, glutamine, and fish oil supplements. She also went on an elimination diet to figure out what was triggering her allergic reactions and allow her gut to rest and heal.

In a matter of 3 or 4 weeks, the eczema began to improve. She began to add a daily dose of "greens" to her diet in the form of smoothies and juices. She also incorporated chia seeds, goji berries, maca, and other "superfoods" into her diet. Her energy levels increased as her micronutrient intake and absorption rates increased.

If you feel like you have lost your health, all hope is not lost. Health can be restored and the gut can heal itself. It takes time and patience. If you start to experience this, it's important to drink plenty of water and cut back your probiotics to once a day until the symptoms subside.

When the Diet Isn't Working

If several weeks have gone by and you're not noticing results, it's time to take inventory of what you're doing and decide on your next steps. First, you need to evaluate your current efforts. Here's a checklist of questions to answer honestly.

Are you:

- ❏ Eating three balanced meals daily comprised of healthy fats, carbs, and proteins?
- ❏ Following the recommendations for neutral foods before introducing triggers?
- ❏ Introducing triggers one at a time for 1 week and tracking results?
- ❏ Keeping a food diary and recording symptoms?

❑ Troubleshooting based on the food diary (for example: limiting FODMAP foods based on GI symptoms)?

❑ Introducing bone broths?

❑ Eating fermented foods or taking a high-quality probiotic (and if excessive gas occurs, reducing the amount)?

❑ Finding time to engage in moderate exercise at least three times a week?

❑ Getting 8 hours of sleep a night?

❑ Incorporating some kind of stress management into your routine (such as meditation, a few minutes of quiet breathing, a hot bath, etc.)?

If you can honestly say you've done all of those things *consistently* for at least a couple of weeks straight, and you're still experiencing negative GI or autoimmune symptoms, it's time for further evaluation.

Prolonged Negative Symptoms

So you've kept a food diary with precision and consistency. You've eaten healthy foods, taken probiotics, and basically done all the right things. And yet you still have unresolved symptoms. You most likely have a brain-gut axis disturbance that isn't responding to the protocol. Take heart. There are some routes you can try.

You can try eliminating *histamines* from your diet. Histamines are neurotransmitters that help us with digestion and immune system function. One of their jobs is to cause an inflammatory response, which triggers the immune system that an invader is present. (We discussed histamines in Chapter 7 when we reviewed health issues involving inflammatory responses, allergies, and respiratory conditions.)

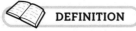 **DEFINITION**

> **Histamines** are neurotransmitters released by your body's cells after an injury. They cause inflammation by inducing the contraction of smooth muscles in your organs and dilation of capillaries.

What makes histamine problematic is that it can cause issues that fly under the diagnosis radar. Asthma and seasonal and food allergies brought about by histamine intolerances in the body can be obvious to you and your doctors. Sometimes, however, histamine intolerance can be caused by a lack of certain enzymes, GI bleeding, or foods that aren't part of the "usual suspects" list for food reactions.

Some common symptoms of histamine intolerance include severe headaches, trouble falling and staying asleep, high blood pressure, vertigo and dizziness, abnormal heartbeat, feeling too hot or too cold, anxiety, nausea (even to the point of vomiting), stomach cramps, nasal congestion, sneezing, shortness of breath, hives, fatigue, and irregular menstruation. While some of those symptoms might seem vague, if you suffer from a combination of any of them concurrently, you might have a histamine intolerance. If you and your doctor have ruled out GI bleeding and enzyme deficiencies (such as *diamine oxidase*), you might consider cutting back on histamine-rich foods that could be overloading your system with inflammatory responses.

DEFINITION

Diamine oxidase (DAO) is the primary enzyme that helps you metabolize the histamines in foods. If you're deficient in DAO, your body will display symptoms of histamine intolerance.

Histamine-rich foods include alcohol, avocados, dried fruits and citrus fruit, fermented foods (they have so many health benefits, but they cause problems for a small number of people; you might have to ease off of them and take supplements), mackerel, mahi-mahi, tuna, sardines, anchovies, mayonnaise, peanuts, walnuts, cashews, pickled foods, smoked meats, and spinach.

Some other considerations if you're having persistent negative symptoms is to make sure you're not eating any "healthy junk." Be suspicious of foods in packaging that boasts "added probiotics," "gluten-free," "casein-free," and "all natural sugars." These are still processed foods, and they can be nearly as devastating to your gut as the triggers they're replacing.

You might also want to eliminate all foods in the nightshade family as these can trigger inflammation for some people. These foods include white potatoes, eggplant, tomatoes, goji berries, and peppers (including spices made from them like paprika). People with autoimmunity and irritated gut linings can be especially sensitive to certain alkaloids and lectins that these foods contain. This is especially relevant for chronic heartburn, inflammation, and autoimmune disorders. If you feel you've tried everything else and have been diligent, try eliminating these foods and keeping a food diary to track how you feel.

GUT WISE

People used to grow plants in the nightshade family as ornamental plants but didn't eat them because they believed they were poisonous. It wasn't until the 1800s that people started consuming them regularly. And certainly, for some people, these foods are no good.

After 6 weeks, and after performing sensitivity tests (see directions in Chapter 17), introduce nightshades one at a time, one a week, and see if you react to all or just one of them. While there is no clear cut peer-reviewed study that demonstrates the inflammatory effects of eating foods in the nightshade family, there are mountains of anecdotal evidence from integrative and CAM practitioners that suggest eliminating them is worth a shot.

Seeking Professional Help and Guidance

If you experience prolonged GI discomfort and negative symptoms, it is crucial to seek the help of a trained medical professional in conjunction with a registered dietitian. You need to rule out any major health conditions and also have the nutritional expertise of a dietitian to guide you. Going it alone is dangerous if you have negative symptoms wreaking havoc for long periods.

Testing for histamine intolerances and for major GI disturbances can help ensure your health and safety while you take small strides toward optimal gut health. Persistent negative symptoms are a sign that your body still needs to find the right fuel in the right amounts. Trial and error, a detailed food diary, and a team of health-care practitioners can help you solve the riddle of what you need. Have patience and hope. Review Chapter 4 and assemble your team. It will be easier to troubleshoot your case if you keep careful track of your eating, sleeping, bowel, and exercise habits.

Long-Term Results

Once you've determined the right balance for your gut, you can reap the rewards of long-term health and energy. We've given you the guidelines for the best results. You need to adhere to a nutrient-dense diet comprised of probiotic foods, healthy fats, lean proteins, a balance of starchy and nonstarchy veggies, gluten-free grains (in moderation), and fresh fruits. Don't forget to include lifestyle choices like avoiding toxic exposures, incorporating stress management, and getting exercise and a good night's sleep.

The healthy gut diet is more than just food. It's a lifestyle that will yield many benefits, including a healthy weight and metabolism, healthy skin, optimal cardiovascular health, improved respiratory function, optimal immune system function, balanced microbiota (which helps the entire body), normal intestinal permeability, high glutathione levels to ensure proper detoxing and methylation, less inflammation, less chronic pain, decrease of and even remission of autoimmune disorders, and increased odds of only the good genes expressing themselves and keeping the bad ones dormant. That's all reason enough to have patience if your trial-and-error period is especially long. Some of us require more time to adjust than others.

But there's a solution if you can see it through to the end and enlist professional health of multiple CAM and conventional providers.

The Least You Need to Know

- When you give up unhealthy foods, you help your body's detox processes release built-up toxins that have been overtaxing your system.

- Detoxing your body can produce unpleasant symptoms, but these are usually short-lived.

- Adding lots of fresh vegetables, healthy grains, and fruits to your diet can cause gas and bloating. Keep portions in check and be patient as your body adjusts.

- Prolonged negative symptoms after being on the healthy gut diet could be the result of brain-gut axis problems or histamine intolerance.

- Any prolonged negative symptoms should be evaluated by your professional health-care team and a dietitian.

CHAPTER 17

Transitioning

Some gut healing protocols, such as GAPS and the SCD suggest you only need to stick to their regimens for several months up to 2 years. But no gut healing protocol endorses a return to processed foods. These are guaranteed to reinjure the gut lining, disrupt the gut microbe population, and eventually cause a leaky gut all over again.

In this chapter, we discuss how you know when you can indulge in foods you've given up. Be prepared, however, there might be some trigger foods you can never eat again without unpleasant immune or GI responses. Everyone's personal chemistry is unique. You'll have different levels of tolerance for foods, and you'll have to gauge what's going to work for you. We show you how.

In This Chapter

- When, and, if transitioning to a "normal" diet is feasible
- How to safely reintroduce trigger foods
- How to conduct a sensitivity test
- Tracking your symptoms
- Troubleshooting long-lasting negative symptoms
- How to know if the healthy gut diet is "forever"

Is the Healthy Gut Diet Forever?

After your intestinal hyperpermeability has normalized, the gut lining is healthy, and your microbiota is balanced, it might be safe to indulge in certain foods every now and then. You'll need to read your body's cues carefully and do some personal detective work before reintroducing triggers. You'll also want to ask yourself why you want to reintroduce foods. Try to only reintroduce foods with nutritional value that may have caused unpleasant symptoms for you in the past, such as full-fat dairy, foods high in FODMAPs or histamines, and fermented foods. But try your absolute best to steer clear of processed foods forever.

When (and Why) to Transition

After several months of restriction, you might be feeling great and want to expand your food options. This is entirely understandable. You'll probably even feel like you've earned the right to a treat.

Let us say this, the more severe your GI or autoimmune symptoms were, the longer you should try to wait before transitioning to a "normal" diet. What we mean by normal is not the typical diet high in sodium, trans fat, refined sugar, empty carbs, and low-nutrient foods. If you value your health, you'll never go back to eating like that again. It will only put you back at square one while you wait for your immune system, GI tract, and microbiota to revert to the chaos they suffered before you took control of the situation.

 YOU ARE WHAT YOU EAT

One of the hidden dangers in processed food is that they're very easy to physically eat, swallow, and convert into energy. That might sound good, but because they're poor in nutrients, your body will still be hungry again about an hour later. You burn up more calories eating whole foods and digesting them. There's more of a metabolic balance with them. Processed foods go down too easily with little to no nutritional reward.

Your gut lining and microbiota were probably in serious disarray before you started on your journey. You've either healed them or are very close to healing them when you became symptom-free. You don't want to sabotage your hard-won efforts over a bowl of ice cream. Stay strong and slowly expand your diet to include items like full-fat dairy, gluten-free grains, the occasional gluten if you can tolerate it, legumes, and other FODMAP foods.

Reintroduce Triggers and Conduct a Sensitivity Test

If you found there were foods that caused topical reactions, such as eczema, exacerbated asthma, aggravated autoimmune symptoms, or GI problems, tread carefully when reintroducing these triggers. Here are directions for conducting a wrist sensitivity test.

Before eating a former trigger:

1. Wipe a small smear of the food on the inside of your wrist at bedtime.

2. Make sure you use a smear of the food in the state you intend to eat it, as the chemical structures of foods vary depending on how and if they're cooked.

3. If the food is a solid (like a meat), you can mash it up with water first and then smear a dab.

4. Let it dry completely.

5. If the spot looks fine in the morning, try eating a small portion of the trigger.

6. If there is an angry red mark or some other irritation, wait a month and then try the trigger food again.

Only introduce one new food at a time and only one new food per week. Keep in mind that when the gut is recently healed, reintroduction of triggers, especially gluten and dairy, must be done in small doses. Make sure they're non-GMO organic sources. Since dairy is more likely to be better tolerated than gluten, start your reintroduction with those products first.

Here's the basic reintroduction "plan":

1. Choose one food to reintroduce that you have missed the most.

2. Eat that food at all three meals on the same day, but only introduce one new food at a time.

3. For the next 2 days, do *not* eat this food but note any changes.

Your notes during this time will be very informative because food sensitivities can show up even 72 hours after you have ingested the trigger food.

With dairy, you should start with small amounts of ghee and butter, which have little lactose or casein in them, then transition to small amounts of full-fat organic yogurt. After the yogurt, you can move on to kefir and sour cream. Next, you can try organic cheese, but only one variety at a time; cheese has high concentrations of casein, so it might be more difficult to tolerate. With gluten, ensure you try an organic whole grain option, and again only small amounts. Some good examples of gluten-free grains you can try are millet, quinoa, brown rice, buckwheat, oats, teff, amaranth, and montina.

The Importance of Moderation

Even if you're responding well to your newly reintroduced trigger foods, try not to go overboard. It's easy to want to do this when you're tolerating foods and feeling good. But if you overdo it, you run the risk of redamaging the intestinal wall and upsetting your gut microbiota.

Everyone has a limit to how much his or her intestinal lining can take before becoming compromised. Everyone's immune system has a tipping point where too many antigens in the bloodstream signal white blood cells to alert the troops and launch an inflammatory offensive. You want to exercise moderation, so you can enjoy foods but at the same time treat your inner ecosystem kindly. Keep those former triggers to small portions. Hopefully, you'll find that you don't crave them as much as you did in the past.

Tracking Your Progress

When you've dealt with restriction for a long time period and you've reintroduced former triggers successfully, you might be tempted to toss your food diary templates out the window. We're not suggesting you have to document every meal for the rest of your life. However, you do need to be conscious of any old symptoms creeping back into your body.

> **GUT WISE**
>
> Too often, we only consider seeking professional help when everything is going wrong. Even if you feel you're doing great, you may want to consider meeting with a dietitian to evaluate the results you've tallied in your food diary over time. Their expertise can help you obtain optimal results.

For the first several months after you've reintroduced former triggers, take note of how you're feeling. If you notice patterns of heartburn, bowel changes, skin eruptions, joint stiffness, and/or breathing difficulties, it's time to start keeping a food diary again. You may not have to give up the triggers altogether. But you may have some portion adjusting to do. This is especially true of gluten, dairy, natural sweeteners like honey, and legumes. You don't want to tip the scales in favor of microbiota imbalance, increased zonulin levels, and the ensuing problems they cause.

Keep a Food Diary

When you're first reintroducing trigger foods, you need to keep careful track of how much of them you ate, when you ate them, and how you felt in the hours and days afterward. Remember to only reintroduce one at a time, one week at a time. You don't want to possibly overload your system with numerous antigens and risk having a reaction and not be able to track what caused it. When that occurs, you have to start over again and it can set you back weeks or longer.

Putting in the work of record-keeping when you're symptom-free and trying foods again will pay off in the long run. If you conduct a wrist sensitivity test with no negative response, try a small amount of that food. If you try small portions of dairy and show no negative symptoms for a few days, you can increase your portion size. Writing these things down will let you know what are your limits. Keeping careful tabs on your food and your symptoms in the short term is much better than playing guessing games indefinitely.

Track Your Symptoms

This may seem like overkill, but tracking your symptoms is a good idea. At least in the first few months of reintroducing triggers, you should track your supplements, exercise and sleep habits, and stress levels in conjunction with any stress management techniques you use. Here's a hypothetical scenario to show you why tracking this information is useful. Let's say your food diary efforts and observations have demonstrated that you can tolerate 1 cup of yogurt a day with no adverse reactions. Then, 2 months down the road, you have 1 cup of yogurt and notice you're congested a few hours later, or your eczema flares up, or old arthritis symptoms are back. You haven't eaten any other former trigger except that yogurt. You're scratching your head trying to figure out what you're doing wrong.

If you've been keeping a detailed food and lifestyle diary, you might notice some patterns that will help you make sense of "breakthrough" symptoms. That cup of yogurt might have fallen on a day when a major project for work was due, and you stayed up all night working on it so you didn't do your normal workout routine. Or maybe earlier in the week you ran out of cod liver oil supplements and hadn't been taking them for a few days. Maybe you switched brands of probiotics, and the new one didn't have the same variety of bacterial strains, or the yogurt itself was made from a different starter culture.

These are the types of troubleshooting examinations you can slog through when you're faced with resurfacing symptoms. And if your detective work isn't helpful enough, you can always consult with an integrative practitioner or dietitian. Be prepared; they're probably going to tell you to keep a detailed food and lifestyle diary to help solve the problem. You might as well be proactive and do your homework!

Success Story

Hillary C., a client of Wendie Schneider, RDN, LD, MBA

In Hillary C.'s own words:

Two years ago I could not get out of bed without feeling joint pain all over my body. Today, I am a healthy active energetic woman.

I began by working with my rheumatologist and dietitian to start an elimination diet to hopefully help with the inflammation I was experiencing. I eliminated gluten, dairy, refined sugars, nightshades, and packaged/processed foods from my diet. I also made sure the protein I was consuming was high quality and antibiotic/hormone-free. Citrus and bananas were eliminated as well because these fruits disrupted my digestive system.

I saw a significant improvement in the first week alone, and it has continued to improve since. I went from being in complete pain with digestive issues, brain fog, migraines, and insomnia to sleeping 6 to 8 hours a night, and I even went back to work full-time, which I had not done in years.

After a month of eliminating trigger foods, I began to reintroduce foods back into my diet one at a time. After I reintroduced a food, I waited 3 days to see what would happen. I logged my symptoms in a very detailed food log. I found that gluten gave me severe joint and muscle pain. Tomatoes and citrus fruits made my mouth tingle and feel numb. Soy made me so bloated that I felt pregnant. Any corn produce left me achy the next morning, and corn eaten alone made me violently sick.

I was able to reintroduce full-fat dairy and fermented foods like yogurt and kefir back into my diet without a problem.

My story is truly amazing, and my friends and family are so thankful to have me back after being sick for so many years. It is amazing to see how foods affect your body and changing the diet can impact so many things in such a big way. I am truly grateful.

Persistent Food Intolerance and Allergies

Here's another "what if" scenario: what if you've done your homework (tracked your food, your supplements, your lifestyle choices, and your symptoms), consulted with health-care professionals, and you're still having problems? Every once in a while, CAM and integrative practitioners encounter patients who might not respond to healthy gut protocols. This is where a more broad-spectrum and creative approach to finding other underlying causes comes into play. Some epigenetics testing and more trial and error may be involved. And of course you, the persistent and educated patient, need to be at the center of these conversations.

When to Seek Comprehensive Medical Intervention

Make sure you bring up every possible theory and trial-and-error regimen you've gone through with your medical team (and please make sure this includes a dietitian). If you've experimented with low-FODMAP and low-histamine protocols on your own, try doing the same under the direct supervision of a dietitian who can help you navigate the details and give you tips you may have overlooked when you were on your own.

GUT WISE

According to a 2007 study published in the *American Journal of Clinical Nutrition,* between 1 and 8 percent of the population is histamine intolerant, and approximately 80 percent of those affected are women predominantly in their 40s. If your negative symptoms didn't start until middle age and you fit the profile, it's worth getting tested.

Histamine intolerance can be a possible cause of persistent GI problems and autoimmune-type responses despite a whole foods, healthy gut diet regimen. Histamine aids in digestion, as well as communication with the nervous and immune systems. Because histamine travels in the bloodstream, an intolerance to it can affect nearly every part of your body. Eliminating, at least in the short term, foods high in histamines will help you normalize your gut bacteria. (See the list of histamine-rich foods in the previous chapter.)

Since poor methylation can lead to histamine intolerance, your health team may consider ways to support that process in your body. Remember, methylation is the process of passing a chemical fragment made up of one carbon atom linked to three hydrogen atoms. This passing along of molecules aids in the creation of proteins, neurotransmitters, detoxing processes, and even gene expression. When those groups of carbon and hydrogen atoms bind to genes, it changes the way genes express or silence themselves. Methylation is also vital to the production of energy in every cell of your body.

We need the methylation process to make the most important antioxidant in our bodies—glutathione. If we don't have enough of it, our bodies get overloaded with toxins. Without glutathione you can't detox properly and your entire body is more vulnerable and prone to inflammatory responses to histamines, molds, pathogens, etc. If you've been strict in your diet, exercise, stress management, and sleep routine, one of the things your doctor might look at is your ability to methylate properly. There is genetic testing your doctor can perform to check your methylation levels. Once you know what you're dealing with, you'll know exactly how to supplement and adjust going forward.

> **GUT WISE**
>
> People with autoimmune disorders often have low levels of glutathione because their methylation is compromised by mutations in a specific gene called MTHFR. Your doctor can easily test for problems with this gene or test for the elevated levels of an amino acid called homocysteine that occurs as a result of MTHFR problems. Among other measures, treatment for these issues involves supplementing with extra B_{12} and folate. The underlying message here is reach out to health-care professionals. Just because your case is complicated doesn't mean it's hopeless.

Other possible factors for persistent symptoms despite healthy protocols are Lyme disease, mold toxicity, or chronic cytokine issues. Any one of these conditions can decrease the production of a specific hormone, called *alpha-MSH,* which helps regulate the health of the gut mucosa. If you have a leaky gut that doesn't respond to the healthy gut diet or the adjustments in FODMAPs, trigger portion control, or histamines, you may want to ask your doctor about alpha-MSH testing to rule out those conditions, which would have to be resolved first in order to heal the leaky gut.

> **DEFINITION**
>
> **Alpha-MSH** is short for alpha-melanocyte-stimulating hormone. Alpha-MSH functions in your body as an anti-inflammatory and a neurotransmitter that regulates the release of cytokines, pituitary-gland function, and gut mucosa health.

So how do you know if you run the risk for one of these hard-to-diagnose conditions that get in the way of healing the gut? Let's start with Lyme disease and its risk factors and symptoms.

You may have Lyme disease if you have been bitten by a tick and have chronic insomnia, persistent gut health issues despite treatment, chronic joint pain that is unresponsive to other treatments, chronic calf pain, night sweats, and elevated cholesterol. All these symptoms might not happen concurrently, which can make the disease difficult to diagnose. But if you have persistent symptoms like these in multiple body systems, Lyme disease is a possibility. Talk to your doctor about comprehensive tests for the disease beyond the traditional blot test usually used so you can be confident in the results.

Mold toxicity can be another tricky diagnosis. Testing alpha-MSH levels can help identify mold as a problem because mold interferes with alpha-MSH production. Over 95 percent of people with mold toxicity will have low levels of alpha-MSH that lead to a variety of unpleasant symptoms. Possible signs of mold toxicity include chronic fatigue, mood disorders, sleep disorders, immune system weakness, and chronic inflammation. Getting tested and then working to reduce mold in your home and work environments will work wonders for your recovery.

Cytokines, those messenger proteins secreted by immune cells, are also influenced by levels of alpha-MSH. If your cytokines are overactive, they send false alarms throughout your immune system to start the inflammation process even if there's no threat. You want everything in balance. Too many inflammatory cytokines can also damage the gut lining and induce more intestinal hyperpermeability. Again, some blood testing will determine your underlying problem so you can resolve it first and then go on to enjoy all the benefits of the healthy gut diet.

If You're in It for the Long Haul

Everyone's body is different. After you get to the root causes of your symptoms, you may discover that there are foods you will never be able to tolerate. Take heart, you are not alone.

The most common culprits of these food sensitivities are gluten, dairy (cow's milk specifically), corn, soy, and eggs. You should perform your trial-runs with these foods with organically sources ingredients to rule out reactions to pesticides, herbicides, and preservatives. To finally narrow things down, blood tests for these specific antigens can give you conclusive evidence of an allergy or sensitivity.

Gluten especially will raise anyone's zonulin levels and cause the tight junctions between your enterocytes to stay open for too long and cause further reactions to food particles and pathogens. If your body is genetically predisposed to an autoimmune response to gluten, you will have to accept the fact that you'll be eating gluten-free. But since there are so many gluten-free grains and starchy vegetables that are nutrient-dense and so delicious, it will be okay.

Food allergies and sensitivities aside, you may find that you fall into a different "long haul" category. Your gut lining might be more susceptible than most people's gut to being reinjured after eating previous triggers for a while. This build-up of antigens might reach a tipping point in your body and cause unwanted and unpleasant symptoms. You will have to scale back drastically on whatever foods cause these symptoms for you. Again, keeping a food diary is paramount to narrowing down what those foods are for you.

There are so many nutritious and delicious foods that won't cause any negative symptoms for you. The best thing to do is try to adopt a positive attitude to combat the psychology of limitation. Check out all the wonderful recipes we've offered and lists of foods to try even in the most restrictive phases of detox and neutral foods protocols. You will still be able to find variety and replacements for the trigger foods your body can't tolerate. You'll be healthier and have more energy as a result.

The Least You Need to Know

- You never want to go back to eating refined sugar, trans fats, and other processed foods. For optimal gut health, you really need to say goodbye to them forever.
- After being symptom-free for a couple months, you can try your old trigger foods one at a time after conducting skin sensitivity tests.
- Only introduce one trigger at a time, for one week at a time.
- Keep a food and lifestyle diary to record new foods, portions of those foods, symptoms, your supplements, exercise, sleep, and stress levels.
- Health professionals can help combat your continued symptoms. Check for mold toxicity, Lyme disease, cytokine production, and methylation function.
- If the diet is forever, don't despair! There is a world of nutritious and delicious food for you to enjoy that will keep your gut healthy and happy.

CHAPTER 18

Dealing with a Relapse

Even the most diligent among us can slip up from time to time. If you have a plan, you won't feel blindsided or hopeless—although nothing is really hopeless. Even if you have a bad day, a bad week, or a bad month, you can still get back on track. We show you how to avoid those pitfalls and discuss what you can do if you've already succumbed to them.

In this chapter, we remind you of what injures the gut so you can try your best to avoid those behaviors. You learn how those infamous "cheat days" we often give ourselves during holidays and special occasions can be a slippery slope. We review some strategies for getting back on track as quickly as possible, such as becoming part of a group or forum that gives you a sense of accountability. We reinforce the importance of dietitians and integrative medical practitioners, and you'll understand the importance of sticking it out permanently instead of giving in to temptation.

In This Chapter

- What to do if you damage your gut again
- Finding new comfort foods
- Building a multifaceted support system
- Transforming your taste buds for long-term health

Reinjuring the Intestinal Lining

Healing the gut lining can be a slow and hard-won victory. Reintroducing your old triggers successfully is also a time-consuming process that takes diligence and patience. After the gut lining heals, the old triggers you introduced might still chip away at the gut microbiota balance and restart the cycle of damaged enterocytes, inflamed cytokines, and leaky gut. You have to be flexible and adjust and moderate your intake of your former trigger foods.

You might have to abstain from triggers through a second round of detox and neutral foods for extended periods of time to allow for rehealing. However, we don't want you to be afraid to try to reintroduce foods. Tolerance to food will change over time as your gut bacteria begin to get back in balance. Remember to take it slowly, and seek help from a registered dietitian. Most importantly, listen to your body.

When "Cheat Days" Last Too Long

You want to enjoy the foods you used to, especially when the holidays rolled around. Now your microbiota are getting a taste of those sugary, starchy foods again and your cravings are back. Will a slice of birthday cake kill you? No. But one bad misstep can lead to a cheat weekend. Too often that "well as long as we're cheating" attitude becomes the slippery slope to reinjuring the gut lining.

The best thing to do when this happens to you is just start over. That's not to say getting back on track is always easy. But try not to adopt a defeatist attitude and think that because you ate some processed food for a week, all is lost forever; you might as well give up. You healed your gut the first time. You can do it again.

Get Back on the Wagon

No one is perfect. You had the motivation and the patience to start the diet regimen before. Forgive yourself and start again. That forgiveness idea might sound heavy-handed, but a lot of us are very hard on ourselves emotionally when we don't meet a personal goal we've set for ourselves. This negative internal monologue we carry on can have negative physical consequences. Your emotional well-being influences hormonal changes and your gut registers these changes. Your microbiota register these changes and can become unbalanced. Remember the brain-gut axis. Engage in some stress management that works for you.

> 👉 **GUT WISE**
>
> Laughter is an often overlooked stress buster. A well-developed sense of humor can help you see the lighter side of life's trials and tribulations ... even reinjuring your gut. The real-life health benefits from laughter include increased oxygen levels throughout the body, a release of endorphins that boost your mood, relief in muscle tension and lower blood pressure and heart rate (by first raising all three of these and then dropping them, creating a feeling of relaxation), and a boost for your immune system by releasing stress-fighting neurotransmitters.

After you have renewed your commitment to yourself to get your brain and gut in order, simply make your next meal a healthy one and build from there. There's no point beating yourself up over mistakes. It takes time and energy away from reestablishing healthy habits.

What would be productive, however, is practicing mindfulness and acknowledging what led you to eat unhealthy food so you can try to avoid that situation again. Some of us grow lax in our commitments when we're with other people who are eating processed foods. Our guard is down, peer pressure to indulge kicks in, and we feel tempted. Some of us eat poorly when we're feeling stressed. Take a step back and make adjustments.

Make Adjustments Based on Evidence

Examine the circumstances that started you on your slippery slope to reinjuring your gut. When did you first start noticing unpleasant symptoms, and what were they? Did you stop keeping a food diary? If so, consider starting again to give you a sense of consistency and accountability to yourself. Just as you did when you first started your healthy gut commitment, take stock of what you're currently eating and doing in your spare time and make adjustments based on your observations. Take your whole lifestyle and schedule into account.

Here's a "lifestyle inventory" checklist to help you get started:

- Are you taking on too many projects or responsibilities in your life that are making you feel pressed for time?

- Are you making time for mindfulness and stress management?

- Are you making time to plan and shop for cooking healthy meals?

- Are you batch cooking to make things easier for you when you are pressed for time?

- Are you exercising and getting enough sleep?

- What steps can you take to make more time for healthy habits in your life?

That last item on the list is probably the most difficult *and* the most important. What often derails our best efforts is a lack of commitment to ourselves because we let other priorities outrank our health. Try to remind yourself that without optimal health you cannot accomplish everything else in your life to the best of your ability. That includes being a parent, spouse, family member, and career-minded individual.

If your health comes first, you will have more time and energy for everything else in your life and to do it with more zeal than ever before. We all lose sight of our goals, and we all need reminders of from time to time. When you're reevaluating the way you budget your time to make more time for yourself, see if there aren't tasks and responsibilities you could delegate to others at work or at home. Think about how good you feel when you're helping others and give someone the opportunity to help you so they can feel good about being helpful, too.

Avoiding Temptation

Temptation is at every turn. The cakes and treats in the office break room. The interior aisles of the grocery store. The cabinet of junk food your partner refuses to throw away. The entertaining late-night movie that just started on TV right before you were going to be good and turn in for your 8 hours of sleep.

If you've reinjured your gut and are trying to start over, trying to combat a second round of temptation can seem daunting. You might want to get more serious about your strategies. An effective and habit that reduces the temptation to overeat is making the effort to sit down and eat meals at a table. This is another way to practice mindful eating. When you're out and about, continue to be mindful of what you eat.

> **ASK THE EXPERTS**
>
> Willpower may save us in the moment, but only for a moment, and is exhausting. Enthusiasm generated by purpose and meaning, however, is durable, exhilarating, and most positively the antidote to temptation.
>
> —Mark Houliff, PhD, CNC, FAAIM, DCCN, Consultative Health and Nutrition, Brooklyn, NY

The ultimate in resisting temptation is also making a commitment to yourself. Instead of just thinking about how you're going to achieve a healthy gut again, think about why? Think about the value of living an active healthy life with people you love and engaging in activities that bring you joy and a sense of meaning and purpose.

Make Changes Gradually

Introduce one healthy food at a time for each trigger you ditch. Rather than getting rid of all the bad stuff at once and feeling overwhelmed with sacrifice, this more gradual approach might work better for you this time. Appeal to the people you live with to get on board and try your best to completely remove each unhealthy trigger you conquer from your kitchen for good.

When you eat, try to practice mindfulness. You'll be surprised how well this works. Have you ever been to a wine tasting? Approach your mealtime as if you were at one of these events. Take the time to smell, taste, and savor the flavors. Don't inhale your food. Experience it. You can even build a social get-together around trying new, healthy foods.

If social situations were your downfall in the past, have a more serious plan to cope with them this go around. Eat high-volume, nutrient-dense foods before you go out to ensure you're be too full to even be interested in the snacks once you get there. If restaurants were your downfall, you can still eat before you go and then only order a drink and small salad so you can still enjoy being with your friends without backsliding.

And while we're on the subject of friends, let's look at the company you keep. Are you spending time with other healthy people? We're not advocating that you end a friendship with someone just because he or she isn't healthy. We're just suggesting you make conscious efforts to also include and spend time with people whose health priorities match your own.

You can also try subtle suggestions to spending time with long-standing friends in a healthier way. For example, if you've noticed that the time you spend with one of your friends usually involves sitting around and eating a lot of snacks, maybe ask to hang out at a local park instead. If your friendships are deep and open, you could just be completely honest about wanting to change the central focus on food whenever you spend time together. You can even volunteer to make healthier options for everyone to try.

Comfort Food Replacements

Sometimes you just feel like eating foods that bring you back mentally to a pleasant memory or experience. Sometimes you just crave certain foods because they taste good. These cravings can subside once you've healed your gut, but if you've reinjured it, those cravings might be back with a vengeance. You'll need a strategy for comfort foods substitutes.

> **GUT WISE**
>
> Comfort foods have been the focus of many scientific studies in attempts to get at why they are so satisfying to us. Mostly it's the conjuring of fond and carefree memories. The olfactory bulb in the brain that processes smell is connected to the limbic system, which deals with emotions and memories.

When you really want something sweet, have some fruit. Remember the frozen bananas in a food processor trick? It will taste and feel like ice cream in your mouth. Yes, we're serious. Try it. When you want savory foods that are rich and creamy, but dairy has given you trouble, try blending raw cashews or cashew butter into recipes to make creamy rich sauces and soups. You can even mix the cashew butter with broth, almond milk, and nutritional yeast, and pour it over gluten-free pasta for a healthier macaroni and cheese alternative. These substitution strategies can help get you over the hump of craving the unhealthy versions.

Finding Support

One of the hardest things for many of us to do is reach out for help when we need it. We are much more likely to be successful if we surround ourselves with friends, acquaintances, and health-care professionals who will support us in our healthy gut efforts.

We've already examined the value of building a health-care network. If you find yourself slipping and you haven't yet built that medical team, go back to Chapter 4. You need to incorporate integrative health approaches and the help of a dietitian, especially if you're having trouble staying on track. Additionally, let's look at what you can do socially with everyday people to get the support you need. You can use social networking and in-person groups to your advantage.

Online Forums and Groups

If you're a smartphone user and feel the pull of an on-the-go lifestyle, using your quick moments of internet connection to reinforce healthy habits can become second nature. Remember those apps we gave you for food diaries in Chapter 9? Many of those apps also connect you to an online community. Online forums are perfect for asking questions, exchanging recipes, and offering and receiving encouragement. In addition to those app-based communities, there are many more based on specific gut health diet plans like Paleo, SCD, and GAPS. We've collected a comprehensive list for you and included it in Appendix B.

> **GUT WISE**
>
> Having trouble finding an in-person healthy eating support group? Start your own. There are excellent online platforms that help you connect with people in your area who then meet in public locations to discuss and share their common interests. Meetup.com is a great place to start. You enter your zip code and look for local groups you're interested in, and if there isn't one you simply click "Start your own meetup." People in your area might be looking for support and encouragement, too. You can be the "healthy gut hero" of your town.

If you prefer to meet face to face with people in real time to foster an atmosphere of encouragement, start with local places where healthy people are bound to congregate, such as gyms and health food stores. Finding a local healthy gut group can be as simple as going up to the customer service area of a Whole Foods store and asking them if they know of one. These types of stores usually carry the business cards of local integrative health practitioners who often run their own support groups. Additionally, health food stores often host cooking classes where you're bound to find like-minded people on a similar gut health journey to yours.

The Buddy System

Sometimes a group isn't enough. You have to actually get to the group meetings, and that means following through with a commitment you've made to yourself. Too many of us will let ourselves down in ways we would never do to a friend or a family member. If you find yourself always putting your own needs last on your "to-do" list, the buddy system might work for you.

The buddy system for the healthy gut diet is the same as having a workout buddy you make a date with to meet at the gym. Having a partner who shares your mission will give you a sense of accountability. If you don't show up at that healthy cooking class you signed up for with your buddy, you'll be letting him or her down. Sometimes that's the extra push people need to follow through when they're feeling tired after work and are entertaining thoughts like, "skipping just one meeting isn't a big deal."

We're not saying everyone needs to dedicate themselves to outside meetings, forums, and accountability partners to be successful in achieving optimal gut health. But if you know yourself well, and you've let yourself down too many times before and slipped into bad eating habits, try the buddy system and an in-person support group, cooking, or exercise class. Being a part of a group and making it a priority to go there with will bolster your mood and keep you motivated.

Staying Persistent and Consistent

The main takeaway here is the old adage, "If at first you don't succeed, try, try again." We have all tried and failed at something. The difference between success and failure is in a person's willingness to persevere despite setbacks.

Keep troubleshooting your lifestyle and eating choices until you find the balance that you and your microbiota seem happy with. And give yourself permission to take a lot of time with your healthy gut experiment. Chances are, it has taken you many years to get to the point where you researched your problem and some possible solutions. Transforming your habits and your body takes time. Be persistent and consistent and you will succeed.

Taste Bud Transformation

If you've found yourself eating triggers again and are trying to get back into the swing of healthier eating, remember to try new healthier options multiple times. Changing your brain's pleasure receptors to respond to vegetables over MSG, refined sugars, and carbs will not happen overnight.

 YOU ARE WHAT YOU EAT

Have you ever wondered why you crave more sweet foods in your youth? It's all about evolution. Children's taste buds are more sensitive to bitter foods because bitter foods in the foraging world of our ancestors signaled "poison." Sweet-tasting foods in the wild are safe and contain life-giving calories. These sensitivities in children's taste buds last until adolescence. The comfort food trap, however, may lead you seek some literally sweet memory from that time in your life.

When it comes to food, first impressions can be wrong. We often decide whether we like a food or not before we even try it. Being aware of this bias can help us stop the development of food aversions. Challenge yourself to try foods several different ways until you find a way that you like it.

You need to eat a new food approximately 15 times before it becomes something you, your brain, and your microbiota prefer. This is the advice pediatricians give about introducing vegetables to children. We adults can be very much like kids when we're trying something new. Be patient and persistent and your taste buds will change over time if you give them the chance.

The Satisfaction of Long-Term Goals

Continue to remind yourself of the overarching goal of your healthy gut diet. You want to reclaim your health. You want more energy, longevity, and a general sense of well-being.

If you've reinjured your gut, start over. Take stock of your symptoms, bust out the food and lifestyle diary, and get to work. You know what you have to do. You've done it before. Perhaps you'll need to take into consideration that certain trigger foods were too much of a slippery slope leading you to portions that were too large and upset the balance you had achieved. Perhaps you're not managing your stress well.

Set long-term health and emotional goals for yourself and write down a list of steps you need to take to make them a reality. Writing things down makes them more tangible and accessible. It's like making a contract with yourself. Think about how great you were once feeling when you'd achieved gut health. Think about sustaining that feeling. Now go for it.

The Least You Need to Know

- It's never too late to change course. If you've reinjured your gut, regroup, and start over.
- Chart your eating and lifestyle habits and make changes, including how and where you socialize.
- Be honest about your needs for comfort foods and find healthy alternatives for them.
- Make deliberate strides to congregate where other healthy people are and forge relationships with them.
- Join or form some kind of support group to make you feel accountable to your commitment to gut health.
- Focus on the long-term health benefits that outweigh short-lived pleasure from unhealthy food. Stay committed to yourself. You're worth it.

Glossary

alkaline   The term that describes compounds with a pH greater than 7 capable of neutralizing acids.

alpha MSH (alpha melanocyte stimulating hormone)   Alpha MSH functions in your body as an anti-inflammatory and a neurotransmitter that regulates the release of cytokines, pituitary gland function, and gut mucosa health.

anemia   A medical condition in which the ability of the blood to deliver oxygen to body systems has been compromised.

anorexia nervosa   An eating disorder characterized by the patient's refusal of food, distorted body image, and obsession with losing weight.

antibodies   Protein molecules produced to interact with antigens to develop immune responses to fight off foreign invaders.

antigens   Genetic markers on the outside of an organism that allow antibodies to recognize them as invaders, such as allergens or irritants that cause a reaction.

antioxidant   Any substance that counteracts the negative effects of oxidation in living organisms.

ATP (adenosine triphosphate)   ATP refers to the molecule cells produce to store energy they need for all cell functions.

autoimmune disorders   Any of at least 80 classified disease types in which a person's immune system attacks, and sometimes destroys, his or her own healthy cells and tissues.

autoimmunity   The combination of immune responses that result in an organism's immune system attacking its own healthy tissues.

batch cooking   Multiplying a recipe to make a lot of a particular meal or dish and then storing the food in one large batch (such as a casserole or lasagna tray) or in individual portions for later use. Meals made from batch cooking are usually frozen.

B-cells   Types of lymphocytes, white blood cells, which produce antibodies.

bifidobacterium   A strain of bacteria that in healthy population ratios helps maintain the integrity of the intestinal wall.

bile   A yellowish fluid produced by the liver that the gallbladder stores and then sends to the small intestines to help with digestion, especially with the digestion of fats.

bioavailability   The extent to which a nutrient or substance will be absorbed and have an active effect in the body.

body dysmorphia   A distorted body image characteristic of people suffering from anorexia and bulimia.

BPA (bisphenol A)   A compound used in plastics and resins that can be found in food containers.

bronchioles   The smaller airways that branch off the two main airways in the lungs and end in tiny air sacs called alveoli.

bulimia   An eating disorder with all the symptoms of anorexia in addition to periods of binge eating, self-induced vomiting, and fasting.

cardiovascular system   The part of the circulatory system that moves blood through the body: heart, blood, arteries, veins, and capillaries.

central nervous system   The part of the nervous system made of the brain and spinal cord.

circadian rhythms   Biological processes regulated by the internal clock of the suprachiasmatic nucleus in roughly 24-hour-long patterns.

circulatory system   The system responsible for moving blood and lymph through the body; it is made up of the heart, arteries, capillaries, veins, lymphatic vessels, and glands.

cirrhosis   A disease caused by alcohol abuse or hepatitis. The disease affects the liver and is characterized by inflammation, cell damage and degeneration, and a thickening of organ tissue.

clostridia   Strains of bacteria commonly found in the gut. Some are pathogenic, like those causing tetanus and botulism, and some are beneficial, like those that help prevent food allergies.

colonoscopy   A medical diagnostic procedure, usually performed by a gastroenterologist, that detects abnormalities in the rectum and large intestine (colon). It involves the insertion of a tiny camera fixed to the end of a long tube into the anus and colon.

colorectal polyps   Growths that extend outward from colon and rectum tissues. Sometimes they're harmless, but they can be cancerous and should be evaluated and/or removed by a doctor.

complementary and alternative medicine   Health care that includes both conventional and nonconventional (and traditionally non-Western) approaches to treating patients.

connective tissues   The groups of cells that bind, support, or separate tissues and organs; they are made up of proteins such as collagen.

cyclooxygenase 1   Also known as COX-1, an enzyme used to make prostaglandins, it's essential for stomach and kidney health.

cytokines   Molecules that help with cell-to-cell communication; they specifically help stimulate the movement of white blood cells to a site of infection or damage and inflammation in the body.

diamine oxidase (DAO)   The primary enzyme that helps metabolize the histamines in foods. If you're deficient in DAO, your body will display symptoms of histamine intolerance.

dietetics   The study of nutrition and its effect on the body.

dietitian   An expert in nutrition with a degree in science, practical training, and board certification.

digestion   The body's process of breaking food down into nutrients that can then be appropriately absorbed and used.

digestive system   The group of organs working collectively to break down food into nutrients that can absorbed by the body. It consists of the mouth, esophagus, stomach, small intestine, pancreas, liver, gallbladder, colon, rectum, and anus.

disaccharide   A sugar made up of two simple or "monosaccharides" joined together in a chemical bond in which one molecule of water is removed.

diverticulitis   The inflammation of small pouches that line the wall of the colon.

dopamine   A substance that acts as both a neurotransmitter and a hormone. It plays a role in regulating your mood.

duodenum   The first portion of the small intestine (measuring approximately 10 inches) that receives enzymes and hormones from the ducts that lead to the gallbladder and pancreas.

E. coli   A bacteria found in the GI tract of most people. Certain strains in contaminated food can cause major GI upset.

electrolytes   Substances that split into their separate ions in a solution and are capable of conducting electricity. Salt (sodium chloride) splits into its separate components in water and in the body helps conduct nerve impulses and aids in homeostasis.

endorphins   Proteins produced by the central nervous system that act like natural opiates. Your body releases these proteins during stress and pain to reduce your perception of discomfort.

endoscopy   A medical procedure utilizing similar tools as a colonoscopy to examine your upper digestive tract from your throat to your small intestine.

enteric nervous system   This section of the nervous system is sometimes referred to as "the second brain"; it's the portion of the nervous system comprised of tens of millions of neurons and nerve cells located inside the walls of the GI tract, pancreas, and gallbladder.

enterocytes   The surface cells that line the intestinal wall.

enzyme   A substance made by a living thing that aids in chemical reactions like those involved in digestion.

epigenetics   The study of how genes express themselves and what factors influence those expressions.

epithelial cells   The cells that make up the thin surface layer of body structures, like those that make up the surface of the intestines.

FODMAPs   The acronym for fermentable oligosaccharides, disaccharides, monosaccharides, and polyols. These substances are hard for the small intestine to digest. In susceptible individuals, they can feed pathogenic bacteria.

free radicals   Unstable molecules that bind to other molecules to gain stability. This causes oxidative stress, which leads to abnormal cell activity and damage.

gallbladder   The small, pear-shaped organ located near the liver that stores the bile used in digestion.

gastritis   Erosion, irritation, or inflammation of the stomach lining.

gastroenterologist   A medical specialist in the digestive system.

gastrointestinal tract   The line of tubular tissues and organs responsible for digesting food that extends from your mouth to your anus.

gelatin   A water-soluble protein produced from collagen. It's very soothing to the gut.

genes   Tiny structures made up of strands of DNA molecules that instruct individual body cells to make the different proteins they need to form and function. Your genes are inherited and passed on to the next generation.

genetic marker   A gene used to identify a chromosome or other genes that indicate specific traits (like those for certain inherited diseases).

gliadin   A protein found in gluten that triggers the production, and often overproduction, of zonulin in the intestine.

glutathione   A molecule in the body that helps enzymes work in body detoxification processes. It acts as an antioxidant and consists of a chain of three fatty acids: glutamic acid, cysteine, and glycine.

gluten-induced enteropathy   Another term for celiac disease. In affected individuals, ingesting gluten causes small intestinal inflammation, excessive zonulin production, and, therefore, a hyperpermeable intestinal lining. Left untreated, this condition leads to chronic diarrhea, weight loss, and malnutrition.

gut   Another word for your gastrointestinal tract or the part of your digestive system that runs from your mouth to your anus.

gut dysbiosis   A condition characterized by an imbalance in gut microbial populations where there are more pathogenic bacteria than beneficial strains.

gut mucosa   The lining of the intestines, also known as intestinal mucosa or intestinal mucous membrane.

hemorrhoids   Enlarged blood vessels of the colorectal tissues.

histamines   Neurotransmitters released by your body's cells after an injury. They cause inflammation by inducing the contraction of smooth muscles in your organs and dilation of capillaries.

homeostasis   Also called "equilibrium"; the striving of biological systems, including systems of the human body, to maintain a state of balance in which all internal conditions adjust and adapt to change from outside or inside the system.

hydrochloric acid   A combination of hydrogen chloride in water; it's a powerful gastric acid in the stomach that helps break down food.

hypochlorhydria   The term for low stomach acid, the condition in which your stomach and other digestive organs do not produce enough of the gastric secretion called hydrochloric acid.

ileum   The last third of the small intestinal tract; it measures about 12 feet long and is specialized to absorb nutrients, especially vitamin B_{12} and bile salts.

immunoglobulins   Specialized proteins, also called antibodies, produced by your immune system.

integrative medicine   A patient-centered approach to health care that takes into account physical, psychological, social, environmental, and spiritual influences at work in their lives.

jejunum   The middle section of the small intestine that measures about 8 feet long and is specialized to absorb nutrients.

lactobacillus   A strain of bacteria that produces lactic acid; healthy populations of the bacteria help maintain the integrity of the intestinal wall.

lactose   The naturally occurring sugar in milk.

lactulose/mannitol test   A clinical test during which a patient fasts and then ingests a drink containing two sugars that aren't metabolized, lactulose and mannitol, to determine intestinal hyperpermeability.

leaky gut   Another term for intestinal permeability; this occurs when gaps between cells in the intestinal lining allow pathogens and undigested food particles to pass directly into the circulatory system.

limbic system   A network of nerves in the brain associated with instinct and emotions. It controls more basic feelings and instinctual drives like hunger, dominance, parenting, and sex.

lower esophageal sphincter (LES)   The ring-shaped muscle that serves as the pathway from the esophagus into the stomach.

lymphatic system   The part of the circulatory system that moves lymph through the body; it is made of lymphatic vessels and nodes, the spleen, and the thymus.

lymphocytes   White blood cells of the immune system (B-cells and T-cells) that produce antibodies and attack foreign invaders (or perceived foreign invaders) throughout the body.

macronutrients   Life-sustaining substances that include carbohydrates, proteins, and fats that can be more directly used as energy.

mast cells   Cells in the connective tissues of your body that release substances in response to inflammation or injury.

melatonin   A hormone that helps modulate sleep and wake cycles.

metabolism   The physical and chemical processes that take place inside the cells of living organisms; basically its everything your body has to do to convert food into energy.

metabolites   Small molecules produced during metabolism, which includes all the processes necessary for cell generation, growth, survival, and reproduction.

methylation   The process that regulates gene expression and cell repair. It occurs when a set of one carbon linked to three hydrogen molecules is given to a molecule.

microbes   Tiny organisms such as the bacteria (both beneficial and pathogenic) that live in the human GI tract.

microbiome   The community of microorganisms living together in a particular environment, including the body.

micronutrients   Life-sustaining substances that include vitamins and minerals; these serve as catalysts in the body's chemical reactions that influence the release of energy in macronutrients.

monounsaturated fats   Fats containing only one double bond in each of their molecules; these are the fats associated with lower "bad" cholesterol.

neurotransmitters   Chemicals in the nervous system that send signals between nerve cells or from the nervous to other systems in the body.

nutrients   Substances containing nourishment crucial in maintaining life.

nutritionist   A person who has completed coursework in nutrition; the title, however, is not accredited. Nutritionists may have degrees in food science or nutrition, but they are not required to undergo accredited practical training in a medical environment and are not qualified to diagnose or treat diseases.

oligosaccharides   Carbohydrates whose molecules are generally made of between 3 and 10 monosaccharides. Oligosaccharides are often referred to a prebiotic food for bacteria.

organ   A group of similar tissues combined to work together as one unit for a certain specialized function in a living organism.

oxtail   The tail of an ox or any cattle. When cooked for long periods, oxtail falls off the bone and provides nutritious gelatin for your bone broth or stock.

pancreas   The glandular organ located behind the stomach between the upper small intestine and the spleen. The pancreas secretes enzymes and hormones critical in digestion and blood sugar regulation.

pathogen   A disease-causing agent that infects or brings harm to its host organism.

peripheral nervous system   The network of nerves throughout the body that are outside your spinal column and brain and connect the rest of your body to the central nervous system.

peripheral neuropathy   The weakness, burning or stabbing pain, and/or numbness primarily in the hands and feet or elsewhere in the body that occur as the result of nerve damage.

peristalsis   The series of involuntary muscular contractions along the gastrointestinal tract that work to propel the contents of the gut forward.

Peyer's patches   Bundles of nerve tissue on the intestinal wall that communicate with antigens in the intestine and send signals to the immune system.

pharynx   The tubular organ behind the nose and mouth that connects them to the esophagus.

phytates   Compounds in legumes and grains that bind to essential minerals, making it difficult for the enterocytes to absorb them.

phytonutrients   Substances found in certain plants that promote health and may even prevent disease.

plasma membrane   The thin tissue layer that lines a body or tubular organ cavity or the dividing space between or within organs.

polyols   Carbohydrates whose molecular structure is similar to both sugar and alcohol, which is why they're often referred to as "sugar alcohols." Polyols are used as sweeteners and include sorbitol, mannitol, and xylitol.

polysaccharides   Sugars comprised of longer chains of three of more monosaccharides.

polyunsaturated fats   Fats with two or more double bonds in their molecules; they are present in nuts, seeds, fish, algae, and leafy greens.

prebiotic   A substance that serves as a nutrient to bacteria.

probiotics   Bacteria beneficial to health, especially those that fight off pathogens.

prostaglandins   Substances in your body that act like hormones and help modulate inflammation.

pyloric sphincter   The ring-shaped muscle that serves as the pathway from the stomach into the first section of the small intestine (the duodenum).

saliva   A watery substance secreted by salivary glands that contains enzymes (like amylase), which helps break down starches into simple sugars.

salivary glands   Structures in the mouth that secrete saliva, which helps break down starches in the first stage of digestion.

serotonin   A neurotransmitter produced in that brain and intestine that plays a role in mood and pain perception.

suprachiasmatic nucleus   A relatively small group of cells in the hypothalamus of the brain that controls the sleep/wake cycles and circadian rhythms.

system   A group of organs working in conjunction with one another with common goals and connected functions such as the digestive system.

T-cells   Types of lymphocytes, white blood cells, that help identify foreign invaders in the body and activate and deactivate other immune cells.

tight junction   The point at which the outer layer of the cell membranes of adjacent epithelial cells fuse together; this reduces the ability of large molecules to pass between the cells (especially pathogens and undigested food particles from the intestinal epithelial layer to the circulatory system).

tissues   Collections of similarly structured cells in an organism.

trachea   The tubular organ in your throat that brings air in and out of the lungs.

trans fats   Man-made compounds produced by using heavy metals to get hydrogen atoms to bind to vegetable oils. They raise cholesterol levels and cause other damage to the body.

ureters   Tubes that carry urine from the kidneys to the urinary bladder.

urethra   The passageway, or duct, that voids urine from the body. In males, this duct also conducts sperm.

urinary system   The bodily system made of the kidneys, ureters, urinary bladder, and urethra that filters, collects, and eliminates waste products from the blood in the form of urine.

vagus nerve   Also called the "tenth cranial nerve," the vagus nerve is a pair of neural pathways that branch out from the brain through the chest and into the abdomen. One of its main functions is to maintain communication between the brain and digestive system.

withdrawal   Any physical or psychological consequences of abruptly discontinuing the use of a substance that has the ability to produce a physical dependence. Some examples include illicit drugs, caffeine, alcohol, and even processed foods.

zonulin   A protein that controls the opening and closing of tight junctions in the gut lining.

Resources

We compiled some books, websites, and support groups to help you navigate your healthy gut journey, find the help you need, and help you feel your best.

Books

Here are some excellent books written by gut health experts.

Blaser, Martin J. *Missing Microbes: How the Overuse of Antibiotics Is Fueling Our Modern Plagues.* New York: Picador, 2014.

Cordain, Loren. *The Paleo Diet: Lose Weight and Get Healthy by Eating the Foods You Were Designed to Eat.* Hoboken: John Wiley and Sons, 2010.

Davis, William. *Wheat Belly: Lose the Wheat, Lose the Weight, and Find Your Path Back to Health.* Emmaus, PA: Rodale Books, 2014.

Fallon-Morell, Sally. *Nourishing Broth: An Old Fashioned Remedy for the Modern World.* New York: Grand Central Life and Style, 2014.

Fuhrman, Joel. *Eat for Health.* Flemington, NJ: Gift of Health Press, 2012.

———. *Eat to Live.* New York: Little, Brown and Company, 2011.

Gates, Donna. *The Body Ecology Diet: Recovering Your Health and Rebuilding Your Immunity.* Carlsbad: Hay House, 2011.

Gershon, Michael. *The Second Brain: A Groundbreaking New Understanding of Nervous Disorders of the Stomach and Intestine.* New York: Harper Perennial, 1999.

Gottschall, Elaine. *Breaking the Vicious Cycle: Intestinal Health Through Diet.* Ontario: Kirkton Press, 1994.

Junger, Alejandro. *Clean Gut: The Breakthrough Plan for Eliminating the Root Cause of Disease and Revolutionizing Your Health.* San Francisco: Harper One, 2014.

Kresser, Chris. *The Paleo Cure: Eat Right for Your Genes, Body Type, and Personal Health Needs.* New York: Little, Brown and Company, 2014.

McBride-Campbell, Natasha. *The Gut and Psychology Syndrome: Natural Treatment for Autism, Dyspraxia, A.D.D., Dyslexia, A.D.H.D., Depression, and Schizophrenia.* Cambridge, UK: Medinform Publishing, 2010.

Weil, Andrew. *Eating Well for Optimum Health: The Essential Guide to Bringing Health and Pleasure Back to Eating.* New York: HarperCollins Publishers, Inc., 2000.

Websites

Here are some great websites for further study on gut health and the wonderful world of microbiota. We also include some links to specific studies and articles that show more of the science behind the healthy gut diet.

Microbiota Overviews

American Gut: americangut.org/?page_id=104

The Human Microbiome Project: hmpdacc.org

Gut Microbiota World Watch: gutmicrobiotawatch.org/en/gut-microbiota-info

Intestinal Hyperpermeability, "Leaky Gut"

The Journal of Nutrition: jn.nutrition.org/content/141/5/769.full

The U.S. National Library of Medicine and National Institute of Health: ncbi.nlm.nih.gov/pmc/articles/PMC1856434

Plos One: journals.plos.org/plosone/article?id=10.1371/journal.pone.0001308

The Brain-Gut Axis

The U.S. National Library of Medicine and National Institute of Health: ncbi.nlm.nih.gov/pubmed/24997031

The New York Times: nytimes.com/1996/01/23/science/complex-and-hidden-brain-in-gut-makes-stomachaches-and-butterflies.html?pagewanted=2

American Psychology Association: apa.org/monitor/2012/09/gut-feeling.aspx

Schizophrenia Bulletin: schizophreniabulletin.oxfordjournals.org/content/14/4/489.1.long

Chris Kresser, MS, LAc: chriskresser.com/the-healthy-skeptic-podcast-episode-9

Psychology Today: psychologytoday.com/blog/the-athletes-way/201405/
how-does-the-vagus-nerve-convey-gut-instincts-the-brain

Scientific American: scientificamerican.com/article/gut-second-brain

Harvard Health Publications: health.harvard.edu/healthbeat/the-gut-brain-connection

Food Allergies

Pacific Standard Magazine: psmag.com/health-and-behavior/
rise-food-allergies-first-world-problems-67067

Dr. Mercola: articles.mercola.com/sites/articles/archive/2014/09/10/gut-bacteria-protect-
against-food-allergies.aspx

Health Canal: healthcanal.com/disorders-conditions/allergy/54488-gut-bacteria-that-protect-
against-food-allergies-identified.html

Health Care and Preventative Medicine

The Chicago Tribune: articles.chicagotribune.com/2013-03-26/health/
ct-met-heart-nutrition-20130326_1_mediterranean-style-diet-heart-disease-diet-and-nutrition

Dr. Mitchell Gaynor: gaynorwellness.com/role-gut-microbiome

Food and Gut Health

National Public Radio: npr.org/sections/
thesalt/2015/07/01/419167750/a-dose-of-culinary-medicine-sends-med-students-to-the-kitchen

Health Knowledge: healthknowledge.org.uk/public-health-textbook/
disease-causation-diagnostic/2e-health-social-behaviour/effect-health-different-diets

Vitamin and Mineral Absorption

Organic Authority: organicauthority.com/health/healthy-bones-with-non-dairy-sources-of-
calcium-rich-foods.html

Scientific American: scientificamerican.com/article/vitamin-d-deficiency-united-states

Centers for Disease Control and Prevention: cdc.gov/nchs/data/databriefs/db59.pdf

Digestion

The Cleveland Clinic: my.clevelandclinic.org/health/diseases_conditions/hic_The_Structure_and_Function_of_the_Digestive_System

Dr. Stool, hosted by Dr. Anish Sheth, co-author of *What's Your Poo Telling You?* drstool.com

The Jay Monahan Center for Gastrointestinal Health: monahancenter.org/screen/all_abo_you.html?name1=All+About+Your+GI+System&type1=2Active

Mind Body Green: mindbodygreen.com/0-14510/10-signs-you-have-an-unhealthy-gut-how-to-heal-it.html

Gut Health and the Immune System

Today's Dietitian: todaysdietitian.com/newarchives/021313p38.shtml

The American Physiological Society: physrev.physiology.org/content/90/3/859

Nature: nature.com/cmi/journal/v8/n2/full/cmi201067a.html

Journal of Ancient Diseases and Preventative Remedies: esciencecentral.org/journals/natural-childbirth-and-breastfeeding-as-preventive-measures-of-immune-microbiome-dysbiosis-and-misregulated-inflammation-2329-8731.1000103.php?aid=14235

Gut Healthy Diets

Mark Hyman, MD: drhyman.com

Joel Fuhrman, MD: drfuhrman.com

The Specific Carbohydrate Diet: scdlifestyle.com, scdiet.org, and breakingtheviciouscycle.info

The GAPS Diet: gapsdiet.com and gaps.me

The Paleo Diet: thepaleodiet.com

The Body Ecology Diet: bodyecology.com

Fertility and Parenting

PCOS Diva: pcosdiva.com/2014/04/leaky-gut-and-pcos

The U.S. National Library of Medicine and National Institute of Health: ncbi.nlm.nih.gov/pubmed/18458209

Parents Magazine: parents.com/toddlers-preschoolers/feeding/healthy-eating/
probiotics-the-friendly-bacteria

Seniors and Gut Health

Health Day: News for Healthier Living: consumer.healthday.com/senior-citizen-information-31/
misc-aging-news-10/gut-microbes-might-reflect-health-diet-of-older-adults-666682.html

Today's Geriatric Medicine: todaysgeriatricmedicine.com/archive/030209p12.shtml

Aggravators of the Gut

Twelve Wellness: twelvewellness.com/alcohol-gut-health-eating-to-restore-balance

Gut: gut.bmj.com/content/43/4/506.full

Meditation as Stress Management and Means of Healing

Allergies and Your Gut, Dr. Joan Hardin: allergiesandyourgut.com/2014/02/21/
healing-meditation

The U.S. National Library of Medicine and National Institute of Health: ncbi.nlm.nih.gov/
pubmed/24485481

Sleep and Gut Health

British Broadcasting Corporation: bbc.com/news/science-environment-32606341

Chris Kresser, MS, Lac: chriskresser.com/
why-most-people-are-sleep-deprived-and-what-to-do-about-it

Support Groups

These are online forums and message boards concerning gut health. Many also offer ways to
connect with people in person.

Cure Zone: curezone.org/forums/f.asp?f=23

Irritable Bowel Syndrome Self Help and Support Group: ibsgroup.org

Bad Gut, the Canadian Society of Intestinal Research: badgut.org

My Fitness Pal: myfitnesspal.com

Spark Health: sparkpeople.com

The Upper Canada Lower Bowel Society: uclbs.org

The Functional Gut Clinic: thefunctionalgutclinic.com

Wild Fermentation: wildfermentation.com/forum

Daily Strength: dailystrength.org/c/Healthy-Eating/support-group

Record-Keeping and Helpful Lists

In this appendix, we give you some sample diaries and shopping lists to help you plans meals, conquer the grocery store, and more.

Food and Lifestyle Diaries

Here are some sample diaries to help you track your habits and progress. Remember, it's not just about what you ate. You need to track when you ate and drank, where you ate and drank, and your portion sizes. You need to log your supplements and dosages. Record your basic lifestyle factors that play a role in your overall health, too—your stress levels, any stress management techniques you employ (like meditation), exercise, and your sleep habits.

Daily Food, Beverage, and Supplement Diary Example

Time	Place	Food/Beverage/ Supplement	Portion Size/ Dosage	Symptoms (Mental and Physical)	Other Notes
7 A.M.	Home	Organic yogurt	1 cup		
7 A.M.	Home	Cod liver oil	1 soft gel = 114mg omega-3		
9 A.M.	Work			Bloating	Yogurt may cause bloat for me

Daily Lifestyle Diary Example

Time	Place	Exercise	Stress Management	Stress Levels	Sleep (Hours/ Quality)	Other Notes
6 P.M.	Gym	Spin class				
7 P.M.	Gym			None—felt great		
9 P.M.	Home		30-minute meditation			
10 P.M. to 6 A.M.					8 hours of great sleep	Workout makes for great sleep

Meal Plans

When you're planning your meals, remember to imagine a plate divided into three sections to be filled with starchy veggies, nonstarchy veggies and fruit, and protein. Try to plan all your meals before making your grocery shopping list for the week. Most people just plan for dinner, which leaves them scrambling to figure out breakfast and lunch. Don't leave yourself open to temptation; plan ahead.

Sample Single-Day Menu

Monday	
Breakfast	High-quality protein (pastured bacon, sausage) and fermented vegetable scramble, 1 cup bone broth
Lunch	Huge green leafy salad topped with protein (meat/fish/tempeh), 1 cup bone broth, kefir or kombucha
Dinner	Stir-fry with protein (meat/fish/tempeh), vegetables, and coconut oil; 1 cup starch (butternut squash, sweet potato, brown rice, or other gluten-free grain)
Supplements	High-quality probiotic, fish oil, glutamine (optional), digestive enzymes (optional)

Shopping Lists

To help you plan for better gut health, we've provided a shopping list of pantry staples, ingredients you'll want to keep on hand, gluten-free foods, and more. We've provided a long list of fruits and vegetables because people often feel daunted when gluten is one of their triggers, so they need a list of approved foods for meals planning and grocery shopping. You don't have to buy all these items during the same trip, as much of it will go bad before you can eat it.

And remember to have a plan for when you go grocery shopping. First, review your meal plan for the week. Next, look in your refrigerator and pantry to determine what you'll need to make your plan a success. Try to buy organic produce, grass-fed meat and dairy, and full-fat coconut milk as much as possible to reduce the amount of pesticide exposure.

Pantry:

❑ Almond butter

❑ Almond flour

❑ Almond milk

❑ Almonds, raw

❑ Baking soda

❑ Balsamic vinegar

❑ Bananas

❑ Beans, dried

❑ Brazil nuts

❑ Broths and stocks, organic chicken and vegetable, bone broth

❑ Brown rice, whole-grain

❑ Capers

❑ Cashews

❑ Chia seeds

❑ Chickpeas

❑ Coconut, shredded, unsweetened

❑ Coconut flour

❑ Coconut milk

❑ Coconut oil, unrefined extra-virgin

❑ Dates

❑ Dried apricots

❑ Garlic

❑ Ghee

❑ Green chiles

❑ Hazelnuts

❑ Hemp seeds

❑ Honey, raw

❑ Macadamia nuts

❑ Maple syrup, grade B

❑ Marinara sauce

❑ Nori

❑ Nut butters

❑ Olive oil, cold-pressed extra-virgin

❑ Pecans

❑ Pine nuts

❑ Pistachios

❑ Polenta

❑ Probiotics

❑ Pumpkin seeds

❑ Quinoa

❑ Roasted red peppers

❑ Sea salt, Celtic or Himalayan

❑ Seafood, canned or packaged, wild-caught tuna, salmon, crab, and clams, without additives

❑ Sesame seeds

❑ Shallots

❑ Sun-dried tomatoes

❑ Sunflower seeds

❑ Tahini

❑ Tomatoes

❑ Vanilla extract, organic

❑ Vinegar, apple cider

❑ Walnuts

Refrigerator:

- ❏ Bragg's amino acids
- ❏ Fruits, in season
- ❏ Greens, fresh
- ❏ Lemon juice
- ❏ Lime juice

- ❏ Salad dressings, organic, made with cold-pressed olive oils
- ❏ Vegetables, in season
- ❏ Yogurt, homemade or organic, full-fat

Freezer:

- ❏ Acai berries
- ❏ Artichokes
- ❏ Asparagus
- ❏ Bananas, peeled and chopped
- ❏ Batch-cooked meals, like soups, sauces, or casseroles
- ❏ Berries
- ❏ Bone broths

- ❏ Fish, wild-caught
- ❏ Mangoes
- ❏ Meat, organic, free-range whole chicken and chicken breasts
- ❏ Pineapple
- ❏ Tortillas, corn
- ❏ Vegetables, without additives

Proteins:

- ❏ Beans
- ❏ Beef, grass-fed
- ❏ Beef marrow or knuckle bones
- ❏ Chicken, free-range, antibiotic free, cutlets, neck/bones
- ❏ Eggs and egg whites, organic, free-range
- ❏ Fish, wild-caught
- ❏ Fish bones
- ❏ Lentils

- ❏ Oxtail
- ❏ Pastured bacon
- ❏ Sausage, Italian
- ❏ Tempeh
- ❏ Tofu, sprouted
- ❏ Turkey, ground

Dairy and dairy alternatives:

- ❑ Butter, grass-fed
- ❑ Cheese, Kerrygold grass-fed buffalo mozzarella, cheddar, feta, goat/sheep, Parmesan, provolone
- ❑ Ghee
- ❑ Kefir grains
- ❑ Milk, almond, cow (raw if possible), hemp, oat, rice
- ❑ Yogurt, plain, almond milk, coconut milk, Greek, homemade, rice milk

Vegetables:

- ❑ Artichoke hearts
- ❑ Arugula
- ❑ Asparagus
- ❑ Avocados
- ❑ Beets, regular and golden
- ❑ Bell peppers
- ❑ Broccoli
- ❑ Brussels sprouts
- ❑ Butternut squash
- ❑ Cabbage
- ❑ Carrots
- ❑ Cauliflower
- ❑ Celery
- ❑ Cherry tomatoes
- ❑ Cucumbers
- ❑ Daikon radishes
- ❑ Eggplant
- ❑ Endive
- ❑ Fennel bulbs
- ❑ Garlic, garlic scapes
- ❑ Green beans
- ❑ Greens, collard, dandelion, mixed, mustard, turnip
- ❑ Kale
- ❑ Kohlrabi
- ❑ Leeks
- ❑ Lettuce, Bibb, dark green, romaine
- ❑ Napa cabbage
- ❑ Onions, green, red, yellow (whatever you like)
- ❑ Parsnips
- ❑ Pattypan squash
- ❑ Pea shoots
- ❑ Potatoes
- ❑ Purple cauliflower
- ❑ Radishes
- ❑ Rutabagas
- ❑ Shallots
- ❑ Spinach
- ❑ Sweet potatoes
- ❑ Swiss chard
- ❑ Tomatoes
- ❑ Turnips
- ❑ Watercress

Fruit:

- ❑ Apples, any variety
- ❑ Apricots
- ❑ Bananas
- ❑ Blackberries
- ❑ Blueberries
- ❑ Cantaloupe
- ❑ Cherries
- ❑ Dates
- ❑ Figs
- ❑ Grapes
- ❑ Guava
- ❑ Honeydew
- ❑ Kiwi

- ❑ Lemons
- ❑ Mangoes
- ❑ Nectarines
- ❑ Oranges
- ❑ Papaya
- ❑ Peaches
- ❑ Pears
- ❑ Plums
- ❑ Pomegranates
- ❑ Raspberries
- ❑ Strawberries
- ❑ Tangerines
- ❑ Watermelon

Herbs and spices:

- ❑ Basil
- ❑ Bay leaves
- ❑ Black peppercorns
- ❑ Chives
- ❑ Cilantro
- ❑ Coriander
- ❑ Crushed red pepper flakes
- ❑ Cumin
- ❑ Curry powder
- ❑ Dill
- ❑ Dried chile peppers
- ❑ Garam masala

- ❑ Garlic
- ❑ Gingerroot
- ❑ Lavender buds (optional)
- ❑ Mint
- ❑ Parsley
- ❑ Rosemary
- ❑ Sea salt
- ❑ Tarragon
- ❑ Thyme
- ❑ Truffle salt (optional)
- ❑ Turmeric

Condiments and oils:

- ❏ Bone broth
- ❏ Butter, Kerrygold grass-fed
- ❏ Coconut aminos
- ❏ Coconut oil, cold-pressed, extra-virgin
- ❏ Fermented vegetables
- ❏ Guacamole, homemade
- ❏ Hot sauce
- ❏ Hummus, homemade
- ❏ Maple syrup, grade B
- ❏ Marinara sauce, Trader Joe's Basil Marinara
- ❏ Mustard, Dijon, spicy, yellow
- ❏ Olive oil, cold-pressed, extra-virgin
- ❏ Olives
- ❏ Red Thai chile paste
- ❏ Salsa, homemade
- ❏ Spaghetti sauce, Eden Farms
- ❏ Tamari
- ❏ Truffle olive oil (optional)
- ❏ Vinegar, apple cider (raw), balsamic, red wine
- ❏ White miso paste
- ❏ Wine, white cooking

Gluten-free:

- ❏ Amaranth
- ❏ Bread, high-fiber, gluten-free (Food for Life Brown Rice Bread, Udi's Whole Grain)
- ❏ Buckwheat
- ❏ Cereal, Nature's Path Whole O's (gluten-free)
- ❏ Crackers, high-fiber, gluten-free
- ❏ Millet
- ❏ Oatmeal, rolled or steel-cut
- ❏ Pasta, brown rice, quinoa, lentil
- ❏ Quinoa flakes, gluten-free
- ❏ Rice, brown, wild, basmati
- ❏ Rolled oats, Bob's Red Mill Gluten Free

Superfoods:

- ❏ Bee pollen
- ❏ Cacao nibs, raw
- ❏ Cacao powder, raw
- ❏ Coconut, unsweetened, shredded
- ❏ Dark chocolate (70%)
- ❏ Flour, almond, coconut, brown rice, nut
- ❏ Goji berries, dried
- ❏ Maca
- ❏ Spirulina/chlorella

Sweets:

❑ Cacao powder, raw

❑ Chocolate chips, dark

❑ Coconut butter

❑ Coconut palm sugar

❑ Ice cream/pops, coconut

❑ Nutiva Coconut Manna

❑ Righteously Raw Bars

❑ Sugar, date

Snacks:

❑ Corn chips, Trader Joe's Organic Corn Chips

❑ Crackers, Mary's Gone Crackers (onion, rosemary, plain, or black pepper)

❑ Popcorn, Trader Joe's Organic Popcorn with Olive Oil

Beverages:

❑ Juices, cold-pressed

❑ Kombucha

❑ Tea, ginger, green, herbal chamomile, liver-supporting (milk thistle, dandelion, etc.), oolong white, peppermint, red rooibos, rose hip, turmeric tea

❑ Water, filtered, infused

Index

E

table salt, 164
trans fats, 164
tracking progress, 250
food diaries, 251
symptoms, 251-252
trans fats
adverse effects, 77
eliminating from diet, 164
processed foods, 89-90
transitioning process
food intolerances and allergies, 252
long-term expectations, 255
seeking medical intervention, 253-255
reintroducing trigger foods, 249-250
sensitivity tests, 249-250
time frames, 248
tracking progress, 250
food diaries, 251
symptoms, 251-252
travel, adverse effects, 34
triclosan, 190
triethanolamine, 190
triggers, foods
eliminating from diet, 129-130
gut homeostasis, 40-41
reintroducing (transitioning process), 249-250
typical diet problems, 81
dairy products, 85-86
gluten, 82-83
grains, 83
legumes, 84-85
sodium intake, 79-81
sugars, 86-87
Tub Cleanser recipe, 187
Turnip, Leek, and Cauliflower Bisque recipe, 230
type 1 diabetes, 28

typical diet problems, 76
dairy products, 85-86
empty calories, 76-77
gluten, 82-83
grains, 83
lack of fiber, 78-79
legumes, 84-85
processed foods
acrylamides, 90
GMOs, 90-91
refined sugars, 88
trans fats, 89-90
sedentary lifestyles, 78
sodium intake, 79-81
sugars, 86-87

U

ulcerative colitis, 95
ulcers, 94
unhealthy gut signs, 17
abnormal digestion, 18-21
acid reflux, 19
allergies, 99-100
antibiotic use, 24-25
autoimmune disorders, 27-28, 97-98
bloating and gassiness, 18
bowel movement patterns, 20-21
digestion disorders
diverticulitis, 95
gallstones, 94
GERD (gastroesophageal reflux disease), 94
IBD (inflammatory bowel disease), 95-96
IBS (irritable bowel syndrome), 95
ulcers, 94

eating disorders, 101-102
energy and weight issues, 96-97
food allergies, 25-26
medical care recommendations, 44-46
gastroenterologist , 48-49
integrative medicine, 50-52
medical testing, 53-57
nutritionists and dietitians, 49-50
personal trainers, 52-53
primary care physicians, 47-48
mental health issues, 21, 102
emotional disorders, 103-104
extreme mental illnesses, 104-105
learning disorders, 106-108
respiratory disorders, 101
SIBO (small intestinal bacterial overgrowth), 18
skin disorders, 26-27, 98-99
symptoms, 45
vitamin deficiencies, 21-24
urinary system, 7

V

vagus nerve, 11-12
vegan diets
dietary recommendations, 158
principles, 158
Vegetable Broth recipe, 214
vegetables
Fermented Vegetables recipe, 217
food recommendations, 165
Grilled Garlic Scapes recipe, 223